Count Your Calories

I0116798

POOJA MALHOTRA

SHREE

Shree Book Centre
98/B, Dalmia Bldg, Opp Sandesh Hotel,
T.H. Kataria Marg, Matunga (W), Mumbai-400 016 (INDIA)
Tel: 24377516, 24374559 Fax: 24309183
Email: shreebk@vsnl.com

Published by Sterling Publishers Pvt. Ltd., New Delhi-110020.
Lasertypeset by Vikas Compographics, New Delhi-110020.
Printed at Sai Early Learners Pvt. Ltd., New Delhi-110020.

Contents

Introduction

Most of us enjoy the food we eat — the variety of tastes that different cuisines have. However, food performs important functions in the body other than pampering our taste buds, and is essential for survival, growth, reproduction and for maintaining good health. As a popular saying goes, 'Don't live to eat, eat to live'.

Food is the 'fuel' which supplies chemical energy to our body to support daily activities and growth. Even fully grown adults require energy for survival, maintenance and repair of worn out tissues. The energy value of food is measured in heat units called calories.

Besides energy, food supplies our body with proteins, carbohydrates, fats, vitamins, minerals and fibre. All these nutrients are required by our body in specific amounts. An imbalanced intake, that is, deficiency or excess, of any of these nutrients including energy, can impair health.

What is a calorie?

A calorie is a unit of measurement of energy. By definition, a calorie is the amount of heat energy required to raise the temperature of one gram of water by 1° Celsius, specifically from 14.5° C to 15.5° C. The new unit of energy, which has been accepted by the International Union of Sciences and the International

Union of Nutritional Sciences, is 'Joule'. One calorie is equal to 4.184 Joules (symbol 'J').

The kilocalorie, which is equal to 1000 calories, is the unit commonly used for measuring the amount of energy which food provides. For all practical purposes, 'calorie' continues to be widely used for measuring energy content of foodstuffs and for estimating energy requirements of human beings. Kilocalorie will be referred to as calorie (symbol 'Cal' with 'C' in Capital), hereafter.

What calories do

Calories provide the fuel to keep the human body going. They provide our body with the energy that we require to perform all our body functions. We require energy for survival – to breathe, pump blood and for all kinds of physical activity like walking, running, sitting and working. Calories are required even when we are lying down or asleep. They are also expended in digestion of food, and for making available the calories from that food to our body. They are essential for maintenance of our body temperature. Thus, adults require calories mainly for physical activities and involuntary body functions. In case of infants and children in their growing years, besides the above mentioned roles, calories perform the very vital function of supporting growth and development.

Your Caloric Needs

Energy is required by all individuals for survival, growth and maintenance but energy requirements of different individuals are different. These requirements are based on three factors:

- **Basal or resting metabolic rate,** which is the amount of energy required by your body to carry out vital body functions at rest. This accounts for about 55 per cent of total calories burnt in a day and includes the energy expenditure in activities such as respiration, blood circulation, functioning of kidneys, maintenance of body temperature and so on. Basal energy or basal metabolism is thus the energy expended by your body in a state of complete rest (both physical and mental).
- **Thermic effect of food** is the amount of energy that your body requires for digestion of food and absorption of nutrients. It also includes the stimulating effect of these nutrients on body metabolism.
- Energy required for **physical activity**, the second largest component of your total daily energy expenditure, varies greatly depending on the type of occupation, and thus on your activity level. Physical activity includes everything from making your bed to jogging, walking, sitting, bending, moving

around, and even moving your finger or batting your eyelid. At this moment, you are also burning calories as you read through the pages of this book, while sitting or lying comfortably.

For any given activity, the total number of calories that you burn will depend upon your body weight. The greater your body weight, the more calories you burn in performing the same activity. For example, a person weighing 60 kg would expend 6 Cal per minute in swimming whereas a person weighing 80 kg would expend 8 Cal per minute in the same exercise.

Energy expenditure in any activity also depends upon the intensity with which the activity is performed. For example, a person weighing 60 kg will burn 10 Cal per minute while running at 6 miles per hour. The same individual will burn 13 Cal per minute in running at 7.5 miles per hour and 17 Cal per minute at 10 miles per hour.

Although there is a large variation from individual to individual in occupational activity, for the sake of computation, occupations have been classified as sedentary, moderate and heavy. To find out your activity level, refer to the *Know your activity level* box.

Know your activity level

Sedentary
 Male:
 Teacher, Tailor, Barber, Executive, Businessman, Shoemaker, Priest, Retired Personnel, Landlord, Peon, Postman, etc.
 Female:
 Teacher, Tailor, Executive, Businesswoman, Housewife, Nurse, etc.
Moderate
 Male:
 Fisherman, Basket-maker, Potter, Goldsmith, Agricultural labourer, Carpenter, Mason, Rickshaw-puller, Electrician,

Fitter, Turner, Welder, Industrial labourer, Coolie, Weaver, Driver, etc.

Female:

Maid servant, Coolie, Basket-maker, Weaver, Agricultural labourer, etc.

Heavy

Male:

Stonecutter, Blacksmith, Mine-worker, Woodcutter, Gangman, etc.

Female:

Stonecutter

Source: Indian Council of Medical Research, 1996 (Reprint)

In case of growing children, calories are also required for growth and building body tissues. The total number of calories that your body needs in a day is the sum of the factors mentioned above.

The calorie requirements of an individual also depend upon his/her age, sex, height, weight, body frame, physiological conditions (such as pregnancy, lactation), and the activity level (such as sedentary, moderate and heavy). Refer to the following table *Recommended dietary allowances for Indians* to find out your daily requirements of energy, protein and fat.

Recommended Dietary Allowances for Indians

Group	Particulars	Body weight (kg)	Net energy (Cal/day)	Protein (g/day)(g/day)	Fat (g/day)
Man	Sedentary work	60	2425	60	20
	Moderate work	60	2875	60	20
	Heavy work	60	3800	60	20
Woman	Sedentary work	50	1875	50	20
	Moderate work	50	2225	50	20
	Heavy work	50	2925	50	20
Woman	Pregnant	50	+300	+15	30
	Lactation (0-6 months)	50	+550	+25	45
	Lactation (0-12 months)	50	+400	+18	45
Infants	0-6 months	5.4	108/kg	2.05/kg	–
	6-12 months	8.6	98/kg	1.65/kg	–
Children	1-3 years	12.2	1240	22	25
	4-6 years	19.0	1690	30	25
	7-9 years	26.9	1950	41	25

Group	Particulars	Body weight (kg)	Net energy (Cal/day)	Protein (g/day)(g/day)	Fat (g/day)
Boys	10-12 years	35.4	2190	54	25
Girls	10-12 years	31.5	1970	57	25
Boys	13-15 years	47.8	2450	70	25
Girls	13-15 years	46.9	2060	65	25
Boys	16-18 years	57.1	2640	78	25
Girls	16-18 years	49.9	2060	63	25

Source: Indian Council of Medical Research, 1996 (Reprint)

The complete summary of dietary allowances for various nutrients as recommended by the ICMR is given in Appendix I.

Food Sources of Calories

When we eat a meal, the nutrients present in the meal are released by the process of digestion. This process begins in the mouth and continues in the stomach and the small intestine. By the chemical activity of enzymes, the complex molecules present in food are broken down to simpler molecules. These simple molecules are absorbed by the walls of the small intestine. After this, they enter the bloodstream and are carried to the sites in the body where they are needed. The simple molecules are oxidised (burnt) to supply energy to perform various body functions. What in the food is the source of those calories?

The components of food which get oxidised to produce calories include carbohydrates, proteins, fats and alcohol. However, one gram of carbohydrate burnt will not produce the same number of calories as one gram of fat. In other words, the calorific values of these components of food differ.

1 gram carbohydrate	= 4 Calories
1 gram protein	= 4 Calories
1 gram fat	= 9 Calories
1 gram alcohol	= 7 Calories

Carbohydrates

Carbohydrates are the human body's key source of energy. When carbohydrates are broken down in the body, the sugar 'glucose' is produced. Glucose is our main source of calories and is critical for maintaining tissue protein. A part of the glucose produced goes straight to the brain and fuels the central nervous system. Our brain completely and solely depends on glucose for all its energy needs. Have you ever felt hungry and found it hard to think? Check out if you have taken enough of carbohydrates in your previous meal.

Glucose is the chief fuel in the body providing 4 calories of energy per gram. This value is less than half the value of fat and equal to the value of proteins. However, carbohydrates are generally consumed in much larger amounts than fats and proteins. Thus, they may contribute more than 50 per cent of the total calories. It is recommended that carbohydrates should contribute 60-70 per cent of the total calories in a day's diet.

Starch and sugars are the major carbohydrates. Common starch foods include whole-grain cereals and breads, pasta, corn, beans, peas and potatoes. *Naturally occurring sugars* are found in fruits and many vegetables, in milk products and in honey, sugar cane, and maple sugar. Foods that contain starches and naturally occurring sugars are referred to as *complex carbohydrates*, because the complexity of their molecules slows down the process of their breakdown to glucose. Thus, complex carbohydrates are digested and absorbed by our bodies at a rate that helps to maintain healthy levels of glucose in the blood.

In contrast, *simple sugars*, which are obtained by refining naturally occurring sugars, require little digestion and are quickly absorbed by the body. These simple sugars are often added to processed foods which tend to be high in fat and low in vitamins and minerals. Such processed foods are thus known as junk foods since they provide empty calories; that is, they are loaded with calories but are devoid of essential nutrients.

Complex carbohydrates are thus far better than simple sugars because of their slow digestion and abundance of essential nutrients. The third reason for the superior health properties of complex carbohydrates is that they contain indigestible *dietary fibres*. Although fibres provide no energy or building materials, they play a vital role in maintaining our health. An intake of 40 grams of dietary fibre per day is desirable. Found only in plants, dietary fibre is classified as soluble or insoluble.

Soluble fibres are found in foodstuffs such as oats, barley, beans, peas, apples, strawberries and citrus fruits. They slow down the absorption of glucose and lower cholesterol levels in blood. They are thus useful for diabetics and help in prevention of hypertension (high blood pressure), heart diseases and strokes.

Insoluble fibres, also known as roughage, are found in vegetables, whole-grain products and bran. These fibres have a significant effect on faecal bulk, speeding up the process of elimination of faeces. Hence, insoluble fibres help in preventing constipation and relieving you from the discomfort and dangers associated with constipation. They also reduce the risk of colon cancer.

Proteins

Proteins are complex nitrogen-containing compounds that build and repair body tissues, from hair and fingernails to muscles and organs. In addition to maintaining the body's structure, they form antibodies (that fight infections), haemoglobin (that transports oxygen from the lungs to the body's tissues), enzymes (that speed up chemical reactions in the body) and hormones (that serve as chemical messengers). Although protein provides 4 calories of energy per gram, the body uses protein for energy only if carbohydrate and fat intake is insufficient. When tapped as an energy source, protein is diverted from the many critical functions it performs for the body.

Proteins are made of smaller units called amino acids. Of more than 20 amino acids that make up proteins, eight (nine in some older adults and young children) cannot be synthesised by the body. These amino acids are considered 'essential' and must be obtained from food.

Animal proteins, found in foods such as eggs, milk, meat, fish and poultry, are considered complete proteins because they contain all the essential amino acids. Plant proteins found in grains and beans, lack one or more of the essential amino acids. However, plant proteins can be combined in the diet to provide all of the essential amino acids. A good example is cereals and pulses. Most cereal grains are lacking in the essential amino acid 'lysine'. This amino acid is abundantly found in pulse proteins which are otherwise deficient in the sulphur-containing essential amino acid 'methionine'. When cereals and pulses are eaten together, these foods provide a complete source of all essential amino acids. Thus, vegetarians must take care to combine cereal and pulse proteins in their diet supplemented with dairy products, nuts and soyabean. *Spirulina*, a blue-green algae, is an excellent source of protein and contains up to 60-70 per cent protein. However, this source of protein has not been widely accepted.

The total daily requirement of proteins for a normal adult is 1 gram of protein per kg body weight (Refer to the table *Recommended dietary allowances for Indians*). Proteins should provide 10-15 per cent of our daily calorie intake. Consumption of large amounts of protein, especially prevalent among non-vegetarians is not beneficial because extra amino acids cannot be stored for later use; on the contrary, they may place an additional burden on the kidneys to eliminate the waste products. Alternatively, deficiencies in protein consumption can impair health by retarding growth and development, and compromising the body's ability to fight infections.

Protein requirements vary with age, physiological status (such as pregnancy or lactation), and stress (such as infection or illness). These conditions place an enormous demand on the body for additional protein. More proteins are required by growing infants and children, pregnant and lactating (breast-feeding) women and individuals during infections or diseases. For example, a healthy woman who normally needs 50 grams of protein each day would require 65 grams of protein per day during pregnancy and 75 grams of protein each day while she is breast-feeding her baby during the first six months after child birth.

Fats
Fats are the most concentrated source of energy in our diet, providing 9 calories of energy per gram; hence our bodies need only very small amounts of fat. They also impart flavour and palatability to our diet which explains why low-fat recipes do not appeal as much to our taste buds as high-fat ones. However, fats in the diet play several important roles. Presence of fat in the diet is important for the absorption of fat-soluble

vitamins such as Vitamin A, D, E and K. Fats, especially vegetable oils, provide 'essential fatty acids', which are important for the structure and function of cells. Fat stored in the body cushions vital organs and protects us from extremes of cold and heat.

Foods in general contain two types of fats, namely, visible fats and invisible or hidden fats. *Visible fats* are fats that are derived from:

- Vegetable fats: Coconut, groundnut, mustard, cottonseed, soyabean, sesame etc., popularly known as vegetable oils. Vegetable oils are also hydrogenated and sold as 'vanaspati' in India.
- Animal fats: Butter, ghee.
- Fish oils: Cod-liver oil

Invisible or hidden fats are those which form an integral part of the foods and are not visible. Almost everything that we eat, as listed below, contains some amount of invisible fat.

- Plant foods: Cereals, pulses, vegetables, spices, nuts, tubers, fruits, etc.
- Animal foods: Milk and milk products (curd, cheese, cream), flesh foods (mutton, chicken), fish, prawns, etc.

Dietary fats can also be classified as *saturated, monounsaturated*, and *polyunsaturated* according to the structure of their fatty acids. Animal fats from eggs, dairy products and meats are high in saturated fats and *cholesterol*, a chemical substance found in all animal fats. Vegetable fats found, for example, in certain vegetable oils, some nuts, olives and avocados are rich in monounsaturated (MUFA) and polyunsaturated (PUFA) fatty acids. As we will see, high intake of saturated fats can be unhealthy and dangerous too.

To understand the dangers of excess intake of saturated fat, one needs to understand its relationship with cholesterol. High levels of cholesterol in the blood have been linked to the development of heart disease. Despite its bad reputation, our bodies need cholesterol, which is used to build cell membranes, to protect nerve fibres, and to produce vitamin D and some hormones. But cholesterol need not be part of our diet. The liver and the small intestine manufacture all the cholesterol we require. When we eat cholesterol from foods that contain saturated fatty acids (SFA), we increase the level of a cholesterol-carrying substance called lipoprotein in our blood that is harmful to health.

Low-density lipoproteins (LDL) and *very-low-density lipoproteins* (VLDL) transport cholesterol from the liver to the cells. As they move, they leave plaque-forming cholesterol in the walls of the arteries, clogging the artery walls and setting the stage for heart disease. Hence, both LDL and VLDL are considered 'bad' cholesterol.

High-density lipoproteins (HDL) remove cholesterol from the walls of arteries, return it to the liver, and help the liver excrete it as bile. For this reason, HDL is called 'good' cholesterol. To reduce the risk of heart diseases, we need to consume dietary fats that increase our HDL levels and decrease our LDL and VLDL levels.

Saturated fatty acids are considered harmful for the heart and blood vessels because they increase the level of LDL and VLDL and decrease the level of HDL. Saturated fatty acids are found in foods ranging from ghee to butter, from cheese to vanaspati. Vanaspati or hydrogenated oil is a saturated fat created by man. It contains saturated fatty acids; and as if this were not enough, the SFA in vanaspati are in *trans* form, which is as bad, if not worse, than cholesterol. Fats containing SFA should make up no more than 8-10 per cent of a person's total calorie intake each day. The total cholesterol intake per day should be limited to 200 mg per day. (Refer to the table *Fatty acid composition and cholesterol content of animal foods*)

Fatty acid composition and cholesterol content of animal foods
(Values in g/100 g edible portion)

Item	Fat (g/100 g)	SFA (g/100 g)	Cholesterol (mg/100 g)
Butter	80	50	250
Ghee	100	65	300
Milk (cow)	4	2	14
Milk (buffalo)	8	4	16
Milk (skimmed)	0.1	-	2
Cream	13	8	40
Cheese	25	15	100
Egg (whole)	11	4	400
Egg yolk	30	9	1120
Chicken	18	6	100
Mutton	13	7	65
Fish (fatty)	6	2.5	45

SFA: Saturated Fatty Acids

Source: Ghafoorunisa & Kamala Krishnaswamy, *Diet and Heart Disease*, National Institute of Nutrition, 1998 (Reprint)

Monounsaturated fatty acids found in olive, mustard, groundnut, palm, sesame, rice bran oils appear to have the best effect on blood cholesterol, decreasing the level of LDL and VLDL and increasing the level of HDL.

Polyunsaturated fatty acids found in vegetable oils such as sunflower, soyabean, corn and safflower oils are considered more healthful than saturated fats. PUFA such as linoleic acid (n-6) and alpha-linolenic acid (n-3) are considered essential fatty acids because these fatty acids cannot be synthesised by the human body and must be obtained from diet in sufficient amounts. (Refer to the table *Approximate fatty acid composition of common fats and oils*)

19

Approximate fatty acid composition of common fats and oils
(Values in g/100 g edible portion)

Fats and oils	Saturated fatty acids	Monounsaturated fatty acids	Polyunsaturated fatty acids		Predominant fatty acids
			Linoleic	Alpha linolenic	
Coconut	90	7	2	< 0.5	SFA
Palm kernel	82	15	2	< 0.5	SFA
Ghee	65	32	2	< 1.0	SFA
Vanaspati	24	19	3	< 0.5	SFA
Red palm oil	50	40	9	< 0.5	SFA + MUFA
Palm oil	45	44	10	< 0.5	SFA + MUFA
Olive	13	76	10	< 0.5	MUFA
Groundnut	24	50	25	< 0.5	MUFA
Rape/Mustard	8	70	12	10	MUFA
Sesame	15	42	42	1.0	MUFA + PUFA
Rice bran	22	41	35	1.5	MUFA + PUFA
Cotton seed	22	25	52	1.0	PUFA

Fats and oils	Saturated fatty acids	Monounsaturated fatty acids	Polyunsaturated fatty acids		Predominant fatty acids
			Linoleic	Alpha linolenic	
Corn	12	32	55	1.0	PUFA
Sunflower	13	27	60	< 0.5	PUFA
Safflower	13	17	70	< 0.5	PUFA
Soyabean	15	27	53	5.0	PUFA

Source: Ghafoorunisa & Kamala Krishnaswamy, *Diet and Heart Disease,* National Institute of Nutrition, 1998 (Reprint)

The total daily requirement of fat is about 40 grams, of which 20 grams is obtained as invisible fat. Therefore, a daily intake of 20 grams or 4 teaspoons of visible fat is needed. Of the day's total calories, PUFA should provide 5-8%, SFA should provide 8-10% and MUFA should provide the rest. An ideal ratio of linoleic acid/alpha-linolenic acid (n-6/n-3) would be around 5:10. To ensure an appropriate n-6/n-3 ratio in Indian diets, the choice of cooking oils should be as follows:

- Soyabean oil which has an n-6/n-3 ratio of around 10.

Or

- Mustard oil which has low n-6/n-3 ratio can be used in combination with groundnut or sesame oil having very high n-6/n-3 ratio.

The quality of fat in the total diet can be further improved by eating 100-200 grams of fish twice a week.

High-fat diets contribute to obesity, which increases the risk of hypertension (high blood pressure), diabetes mellitus and arthritis. Diets that provide more than 30 per cent calories from fat considerably increase the risk of heart disease. High-fat diets are also associated with greater risk of developing cancers of the breast, prostate and uterus. Choosing a diet that is low in cholesterol and fat and hence low in calories, is critical to maintaining health and reducing the risk of life-threatening diseases.

Alcohol
Alcohol provides higher calories (7 Cal/g) than carbohydrates and proteins and thus, can contribute to obesity. Alcohol is a source of empty calories (devoid of vitamins, minerals and proteins) and can be turned into fat, adding weight to the body.

Alcoholic beverages such as whisky, brandy, rum, wine, beer, etc., contain ethyl alcohol (ethanol) in varying proportions (Refer to the box *Ethanol content of alcoholic beverages*).

Ethanol content of alcoholic beverages	
Beer	2 – 5%
Wine	8 – 10%
Fortified wines	
Sherry	13 – 20%
Vermouth	
Spirits	
Whisky	
Brandy	30 – 40%
Rum	
1 ml ethanol = 7 Cal	

Consumption of alcohol in small amounts (a large glass of beer, 35 ml of whisky, or 70 ml of wine) is beneficial for heart; it increases HDL 'good' cholesterol. However, excessive alcohol intake damages the liver (cirrhosis), brain, peripheral nerves, weakens the heart muscle and can lead to nutritional deficiency diseases by suppressing intake. It also increases the risk of cancer of the mouth, larynx, oesophagus, prostate and breast. Also, an initial moderate intake can easily convert into an addiction. Thus, alcohol consumption should neither be encouraged nor recommended for those who are not habituated to it just for the sake of reducing the risk of heart disease.

Calorie Imbalance

All nutrients are required by our body in certain amounts. The energy requirements of an individual depend upon his/her age, sex, height, weight, body frame, physiological conditions (such as pregnancy, lactation), and the activity level (such as sedentary, moderate and heavy).

For most nutrients, an intake level below the recommended amounts can lead to deficiency diseases. However, some nutrients can also be bad when consumed in excess. Energy or calories can prove disastrous when consumed in excess or in insufficient amounts.

The total number of calories consumed, along with the calorie expenditure, has a direct relationship with body weight. When the total calories consumed by an individual in a day are greater than the total daily calorie expenditure, the individual is in a state of 'positive energy balance'. On the contrary, when the calorie intake is lesser than the calorie expenditure, the individual is in a state of 'negative energy balance'. Individuals whose energy intake balances out energy expenditure are said to be in a state of 'energy balance'.

An individual who maintains a state of energy balance over a period of time would also be able to maintain his body weight. A negative energy balance over a period of time would lead an individual to lose some weight. Individuals who persist in a state of positive energy balance would put on weight till they continue in that state.

A proper body weight is most conducive to good health. Deviations of the body weight beyond certain limits from the ideal body weight can have serious consequences besides distorting an individual's body image, general appearance and general health. It can wreak havoc psychologically as such individuals tend to have a poor self image. It also predisposes the overweight or underweight individual to many disorders.

While the problem of being underweight is not new, the problem of excess body weight has come up in a big way with changes in our lifestyle; technological innovations have provided us with gadgets which have made our lives increasingly comfortable and sedentary. With almost everything available at the click of a mouse, we have all become lazy. This has led to a whole generation of chubby people.

What is ideal body weight?

There is no one definition of ideal body weight or desirable body weight. *Desirable body weights* refer to weight for height of young adults at their best physical performance. *Ideal body weights* refer to the weight for height of persons with a long lifespan. Is your body weight ideal? Find out from the table *Standard heights and weights for men and women*.

Another method of determining ideal body weight is given below in the table *Estimated weight allowance for height*.

Standard heights and weights
for men and women

Height		Standard weight				
		Men		Women		
(cm)	(feet)	(kg)	(lbs)	(kg)	(lbs)	
152.3	5′ 0″	-	-	50.8-54.4	112-120	
154.8	5′ 1″	-	-	51.7-55.3	114-122	
157.3	5′ 2″	56.3-60.3	124-133	53.1-56.7	117-125	
159.9	5′ 3″	57.6-61.7	127-136	54.4-58.1	120-128	
162.4	5′ 4″	58.9-63.5	130-140	56.3-59.9	124-132	
165.0	5′ 5″	60.8-65.3	134-144	57.6-61.2	127-135	
167.5	5′ 6″	62.2-66.7	137-147	58.9-63.5	130-140	
170.0	5′ 7″	64.0-68.5	141-151	60.8-65.3	134-144	
172.6	5′ 8″	65.8-70.8	145-156	62.2-66.7	137-147	
175.1	5′ 9″	67.6-72.6	149-160	64.0-68.5	141-151	
177.7	5′ 10″	69.4-74.4	153-164	65.8-70.3	145-155	
180.2	5′ 11″	71.2-76.2	157-168	67.1-71.7	148-158	
182.7	6′ 0″	73.0-78.5	161-173	68.5-73.9	151-163	
185.3	6′ 1″	75.3-80.7	166-178	-	-	
187.8	6′ 2″	77.6-83.5	171-184	-	-	
190.4	6′ 3″	79.8-85.7	176-189	-	-	

Source: Life Insurance Corporation of India

Estimated weight allowance
for height

Body frame	Women	Men
Medium	Allow 100 lbs (45.5 kg) for the first 5 ft. (152 cm) height, plus 5 lb (2.3 kg) for each additional inch.	Allow 106 lbs (48 kg) for the first 5 ft. (152 cm) height, plus 6 lb (2.7 kg) for each additional inch.
Small	Subtract 10 %	Subtract 10 %
Large	Add 10 %	Add 10%

To find out your body frame, pick up a measuring tape, measure your wrist circumference and check out the table *Body frames* given below.

Body frames

Body frame	Wrist circumference	
	Men	**Women**
Small	< 16.5 cm (6 ½")	< 13.9 cm (5 ½")
	16.6-17.7	14-16.4 cm (5 ½"-6 ½")
Medium	cm (6 ½"-7")	> 17.8 cm (7")
Large		> 16.5 cm (6 ½")

Body fat

Besides body weight, body fat and fat per cent are important parameters in evaluating body fatness. Body weight measurement requires a simple weighing machine but body fat and fat per cent are more difficult to determine. A variety of tests are available today. Skin fold callipers can be used to measure skin fold thicknesses at different points of your body such as biceps, triceps, back, abdomen, legs etc. Skin fold measurements are a good indicator of body fat since more than half of the body fat is subcutaneous (underneath the skin).

The skin fold method is somewhat cumbersome and relies heavily upon the experience and skill of the person who is taking the measurements. Electric devices based on bio-impedance and bio-resistance are available now for measuring body fat. These body composition analysers provide a quick assessment of body composition parameters such as body fat, fat per cent, lean body mass (muscle mass), water content and water per cent, besides accurately measuring body weight and computing Basal Metabolic Rate (BMR).

On an average, a normal adult man has 12 per cent of body weight as fat and a normal adult woman has 26 per cent body weight as fat. Accordingly, obesity occurs when the percentage of body weight as fat in total body weight is more than 15 per cent in men and more than 28 per cent in women.

Indices of weight status

Several indices have been concocted for assessment of weight status. Body Mass Index (BMI) and Waist Hip Ratio (WHR) have been identified as reliable methods for a quick appraisal of weight status and the health risks associated with it.

BMI is a measure of relative body fatness. It can be calculated as follows:

$$\text{Body Mass Index} = \frac{\text{Weight (kg)}}{\text{Height (m)}^2}$$

Refer to the box *BMI and weight status* and assess your weight status and the health risks associated with your weight status.

BMI and weight status

BMI	Weight status	Health risk
< 16	Severe thinness	Very high
16-16.9	Moderate thinness	High
17-18.4	Mildly underweight	Moderate
18.5-24.9	Normal weight	Low
25-29.9	Mildly overweight	Moderate
30-40	Moderate obesity	High
> 40	Severe obesity	Very high

WHR is the ratio of the waist measured at the narrowest part between the rib-cage and hips divided by measurement of hips at the widest part. It is a simple but useful ratio. Waist hip ratios higher than 1.0 for men and 0.9 for women are associated with high risk of diabetes and cardiovascular diseases.

Overweight and obesity

Obesity, a worldwide phenomenon, today has surged to become one of the most deadly enemies of mankind, afflicting mostly the rich and the affluent. Obese in simple terms means excess body weight, usually in the absence of an underlying disease, except in a small number of cases where the condition originates from hormonal disturbances.

The terms overweight and obese are used synonymously by the commoner; however, there is some difference at the clinical level. A person can be considered overweight if his body weight is 10-19 per cent more than the normal or ideal body weight. However, when the body weight of a person is 20 per cent or more than his ideal body weight, he is considered obese. As we have seen previously, the ideal body weight for a person depends on his height, sex, age and body frame.

Thus, obesity is a condition of excess body weight and is usually the result of excess accumulation of fat in the body. When energy intake is persistently greater than energy expenditure, the result is gradual accumulation of fat deposits in the adipose tissue depots. Obesity does not happen in a day or a week. It is a gradual process taking place at snail's pace when the individual constantly maintains a positive energy balance. A positive energy balance is usually the result of excessive energy intake. High calorie and high fat foods pamper our taste buds to an extent that most individuals find it difficult to refrain from them in spite of being aware of their nutrient composition. The ignorant certainly cannot be blamed.

The other major culprit is modern urban life-mechanisation and dependence on different tools has made life easy and increasingly sedentary. This has lead to the lowering of activity levels, of daily energy expenditure and thus of our total daily caloric needs. Increased calorie intake due to consumption of processed foods and decreased activity levels have together taken a toll, increasing the prevalence of obesity. Sometimes, of course obesity may also be the result of an interplay of hormones.

Health hazards of obesity

Obesity jeopardizes an individual's health in more ways than one. It imperils both body and mind of an obese individual. An obese individual's distorted body shape and appearance can be a source both of humiliation and discomfort. Many obese people complain of pain in the joints and may develop arthritis (osteoarthritis) because they have overburdened their knees and joints with their excess body weight. This is the most obvious health hazard that obesity invokes.

Obesity has been associated with a wide range of health problems. It contributes to increasing levels of lipids (fat) and cholesterol in the blood (hyperlipidemia and hypercholesterolemia respectively), leading to narrowing of blood vessels due to deposition of fatty materials in coronary arteries (atherosclerosis). This in turn causes the blood pressure levels to soar (hypertension) and increases the risk of heart attack (myocardial infarction) and strokes.

Obesity increases the risk of diabetes because it increases insulin resistance leading to glucose intolerance. Weight reduction helps many diabetic patients in controlling their diabetes. Obesity can also lead to pregnancy related and surgical complications.

Obese individuals are also more likely to develop cancer. Certain cancers such as cancers of the gall bladder, biliary tract, endometrium, ovary, breasts and cervix in women, and cancers of the colon and prostate in men have been associated with excess body weight.

Extreme obesity can also cause respiratory insufficiency (hypoventilation) and may even result in sudden death during sleep. Thus, because of its association with several diseases, obesity decreases life expectancy.

Too much of anything makes you fat
Dietary fat is most often implicated alone in making us fat. Fat indeed is the worst culprit in our diets, but solely counting fat calories is not the solution. Curbing fat intake does not mean you can stuff in all the carbohydrates and proteins that you would like.

Carbohydrates, simple or complex, and proteins can be stored in the body as fat when they are eaten in quantities more than required.

Alcohol is also convertible to fat and all the extra calories from the carbohydrates, proteins and alcohol in your diet translate into fat, which is then stored in the adipose tissue depots in the body.

Underweight

Underweight is most often a problem in underdeveloped nations, associated with poverty, poor living conditions, long term diseases and infections, and ignorance. However, some people, are overly concerned with body weight and have an obsession for a thin body. Such individuals develop a pathological fear of gaining weight and severely restrict their food intake. This behaviour leads to underweight in the concerned individuals.

By definition, a person may be considered underweight if his body weight is 10-20 per cent less than the normal or ideal body weight. If the body weight is less by 20 per cent or more than the ideal body weight, the person is grossly underweight and this becomes a matter of concern.

Underweight is a condition of leanness or thinness and is a result of depletion of body fat stores. When energy intake consistently falls short of energy requirements, the result is a gradual depletion of fat deposits, as these deposits will be mobilised and burnt to supply the body with the much needed fuel - calories. Just like obesity, this condition too takes some time before chronic energy deficiency can manifest as a morbid form of leanness. A long term negative energy balance could be the result of inadequate food intake due to ignorance and low purchasing power, or due to mental illnesses such as anorexia nervosa and bulimia. Increased physical activity, malabsorption, pathological conditions like fevers and hormonal disturbances could also induce or aggravate the state of negative energy balance.

Health hazards of underweight
Underweight results in growth retardation and failure to thrive in growing children. The diet is deficient in other important nutrients such as proteins, vitamins and fats besides calories, leading to deficiency diseases. The result is general poor health and reduced work capacity. The underweight person feels fatigued and listless most of the time. Resistance to infection is also lowered and the underweight person is more susceptible to certain infections such as tuberculosis. Underweight also increases risk of surgical complications and pregnancy related problems leading to preterm deliveries and smaller babies.

Weight Management: Obesity

An ideal body weight is most conducive to good health. It is both preventive and promotive towards positive health. However, as each person is an individual, even normal values of ideal body weight in healthy persons vary over a relatively wide range. Thus, it would be better to define an ideal weight range and also easier to stick to it. The ideal weight range for men and women would be:

> Ideal body weight ± 2 kg

The ultimate goal of any weight management programme is to bring one's weight within the desirable or ideal body weight range and to maintain the weight within that range. In case of obese individuals, management usually revolves around diet modification and exercise, unless there is an underlying disease or hormonal disturbance. The problem of underweight too requires an analysis to seek the causes. Appropriate diet counselling and treatment of accompanying disease form the mainstay of treatment. This chapter deals with the management of obesity; the problem of underweight has been dealt with in the next chapter.

Obesity management

Successful weight loss can be brought about through a combined nutritional and behavioural approach. The food plan should be well balanced and suited to the particular needs of an individual, together with consistent physical activity and exercise for effective results.

I. Dietary management

The objectives of diet modification in a weight reduction programme are:

- To bring about a gradual weight loss.
- To maintain desirable weight and good nutritional status.
- To correct faulty food habits.

To achieve these objectives, suitable diet modifications need to be made.

Energy: Energy intake (or calorie intake) needs to be reduced suitably to meet your individual weight loss targets. A decrease of 1000 Cal daily is required to lose about 1 kg weight per week, and a reduction of 500 Cal per day leads to a weight loss of nearly ½ kg per week.

On an average, a 1000-1200 Cal diet is used for weight reduction in women and 1500-1800 Cal diet is prescribed for weight reduction in men.

How do you decide which weight reduction diet you should follow?

- If you are overweight (body weight is 10-19 per cent more than the normal or ideal body weight), then reduce 500 Cal per day in your actual daily intake.
- If you are obese (body weight is 20 per cent or more above the ideal body weight), then reduce 1000 Cal per day in your actual daily intake.

Another approach for determining energy requirement is based on body weight and activity. Refer to table *Daily energy requirement based on body weight and activity*.

Daily energy requirement based on body weight and activity

Activity	Energy requirements (Cal/kg Ideal body weight/day)		
	Obese	Normal	Underweight
Sedentary	20-25	30	35
Moderate	30	35	40
Heavy	35	40	45-50

Determine your ideal body weight and weight status (by any of the methods given in the chapter 'Calorie imbalance') and your activity level (from the box *Know your activity level*). Now multiply your ideal body weight with the suitable value from the above table to determine your calorie requirement for weight reduction.

Proteins: It is advisable to eat slightly more protein than the normal amounts as protein gives a feeling of satiety and helps to maintain a good nutritional status. Approximately 20 per cent of the total energy must be obtained from proteins as against the normal 10-15 per cent. That is if you are taking a 1500 Cal diet, 300 Cal (20 per cent of the 1500 Cal) must come from proteins. To obtain 300 Cal from proteins, you need to consume 75 g proteins (300/4 = 75).

Fats: Unlike protein, fat intake needs to be reduced for weight reduction. A total of 20 per cent or less calories should come from fat. In a 1500 Cal diet, 300 Cal (20 per cent of the 1500 Cal) from fat will be obtained by consuming 33 g fat (300/9 = 33). The type of fat consumed is important. Refer to the chapter 'Food sources of calories' to find out the type of fat to be eaten.

Carbohydrates: Carbohydrates should provide the remaining 60 per cent of energy. In a 1500 Cal diet, 900 Cal (60 per cent of 1500 Cal) from carbohydrates will be obtained by consuming 225 g carbohydrates (900/4 = 225). The carbohydrates should mainly be in complex form like starches and dietary fibre. Simple forms like sugars should be limited. Dietary fibre (the indigestible carbohydrate) is important to provide bulk and a feeling of satiety.

Minerals and vitamins: Weight reducing diets should provide adequate amounts of essential nutrients like minerals and vitamins, while being low in calories at the same time. Fruits and vegetables, therefore, should be amply included in the meals as they are low in calories, besides being a good source of vitamins and minerals and providing dietary fibres.

Alcohol: If desired, alcohol may be consumed in limited amounts, while taking count of the calorie contribution, that is, 7 Cal per gram of alcohol.

Diet and feeding pattern: The satiety value of the diet is extremely important so as to give a feeling of satisfaction and well being. Adequate amounts of protein foods, fibrous fruits and vegetables, whole grain cereals and pulses provide satiety and thus help to cut down food intake. Increase in fluid intake is beneficial, provided they are not sweetened.

Foods to be avoided:

- High fat foods like ghee, butter, processed cheese, chocolates, cream, ice-creams, fatty meats, pastries, Indian sweets such as burfis, halwas, laddoos, etc., cream soups, salad dressings, mayonnaise and white sauce.
- Fried foods like samosas, mathris, paranthas, pooris, kachoris, potato chips etc.
- High carbohydrate foods such as breads, cakes, cookies, dried fruits, rich pulaos, potatoes, sweet potatoes, honey, syrups, jams, rich puddings and preserves (*murrabbas*, pickles).
- Carbonated and malted beverages, alcoholic drinks and sweetened fruit juices.

The calorie content of commonly consumed raw and cooked foods has been given in the chapter 'Counting calories'.

II. Physical Activity

Regular physical activity is an important part of effective weight loss and weight maintenance. It can also help prevent several diseases and improve your overall health. It does not matter what type of physical activity you perform - sports, planned exercise, household chores, or work-related tasks, all are beneficial. Studies show that even the most inactive people can gain significant health benefits if they accumulate 30 minutes or more of physical activity per day.

How can physical activity help control your weight?
Physical activity helps to control your weight by using excess calories that otherwise would be stored as fat. Since body weight is regulated by the number of calories you eat and use each day, any physical activity in addition to what you normally do, will use up extra calories.

Balancing the calories you use through physical activity with the calories you eat will help you achieve your desired weight. When you eat fewer calories than you burn, your body uses the stored calories and you lose weight. Any type of physical activity you choose to do - strenuous activities such as running or aerobic dancing or moderate-intensity activities such as walking or household work - will increase the number of calories your body uses. The key to successful weight control and improved overall health is making physical activity a part of your daily routine.

What are the health benefits of physical activity?
In addition to helping control your weight, research shows that regular physical activity can reduce your risk for several diseases and conditions and improve your overall quality of life. Regular physical activity can help protect you from the following health problems:

- Heart disease and stroke: Daily physical activity can help prevent heart disease and stroke by strengthening your heart muscle, lowering your blood pressure, raising your high-density lipoprotein (HDL) levels (good cholesterol) and lowering low-density lipoprotein (LDL) levels (bad cholesterol), improving blood flow, and increasing your heart's working capacity.
- High blood pressure: Regular physical activity can reduce blood pressure in individuals with high blood pressure levels. Physical activity also reduces body fatness, which is associated with high blood pressure.
- Diabetes: By reducing body fatness, physical activity can help to prevent and control non-insulin dependent type of diabetes.

- Obesity: Physical activity helps to reduce body fat by building or preserving muscle mass and improving the body's ability to use calories. When physical activity is combined with proper nutrition, it can help control weight and prevent obesity, a major risk factor for many diseases.
- Back pain: By increasing muscle strength and endurance, and improving flexibility and posture, regular exercise helps to prevent back pain.
- Osteoporosis: Regular weight-bearing exercise promotes bone formation and may prevent many forms of bone loss associated with ageing.
- Studies on the psychological effects of exercise have found that regular physical activity can improve your mood and the way you feel about yourself. Researchers have also found that exercise is likely to reduce depression and anxiety and help you to manage stress better.

How much should you exercise?
For the greatest overall health benefits, experts recommend that you should do 20 to 30 minutes of aerobic activity three or more times a week, and some type of muscle strengthening activity and stretching at least twice a week. However, if you are unable to sustain this level of activity, you can gain substantial health benefits by accumulating 30 minutes or more of moderate-intensity physical activity a day, at least five times a week. While including physical activity in your weight-loss programme, you should choose a variety of activities that can be done regularly and are enjoyable to you.

If you have been inactive for a while, you should start with less strenuous activities such as walking or swimming at a comfortable pace. Beginning at a slow pace will allow you to become physically fit without straining your body. Once you are in better shape, you can gradually do more strenuous activity.

Moderate-intensity activity: Moderate-intensity activities include some of the things you may already be doing during a day or week, such as gardening and housework. These activities can be done in short spurts; accumulating 30 minutes of activity over the course of the day can result in substantial health benefits.

Aerobic activity: Aerobic activity is an important addition to moderate-intensity exercise. Aerobic exercise is any extended activity that makes you breathe harder while using the large muscles at a regular and even pace. Aerobic activities help make your heart stronger and more efficient. They also use more calories than other activities. Some examples of aerobic activities include brisk walking, jogging, cycling, swimming, aerobic dancing, ice or roller skating, skiing, and using aerobic equipment (that is, treadmill, stationary bike, etc.).

Any exercise programme should include 'warm up' and 'cool down' periods, each lasting 5 minutes. The intensity of exercise should ensure 60-70 per cent increase in heart rate.

The number of calories burnt during different exercises and physical activities by individuals of different body weights have been given in the chapter 'Counting Calories'.

III. Behaviour modification
Behaviour modification is an important component of a weight reduction programme. It focuses on three components: self-monitoring, stimulus control and self-reward. *Self-monitoring* involves daily record of place and time of food intake, as well as accompanying thoughts

and feelings. It helps to identify the physical and emotional settings in which eating occurs. *Stimulus control* involves modification of: (1) setting or chain of events that precede eating, (2) the kinds of foods consumed, and (3) the consequences of eating. *Self-reward* includes techniques of rewarding self for eating control.

Extreme approaches to weight loss

A desperate desire to lose weight may cause some obese people to resort to extreme approaches of weight loss, which may be undesirable. Listed below are some such extreme approaches:

- *Fasting:* Fasting is a drastic measure and is seldom prescribed as a treatment for obesity. However, individuals often invoke fasting for religious reasons or in a personal effort to lose weight. Fasting may range from total fasting to very low calorie diets (VLCD) providing 200 to 800 Cal. Prolonged fasting can lead to acidosis, hypertension, lowered BMR, neurologic and hormonal side-effects. Fasting is an extreme approach and may be used for very obese individuals strictly under medical supervision.

- *Fad diets:* Weight loss foods available in the market are often based on scientific inaccuracies and may be nutritionally inadequate too. They may infact make weight loss more difficult each time as they may not be practical and may not bring about behavioural changes.

- *Drugs:* Drugs such as ampheta-mines commonly used to suppress appetite may cause many side effects. Phenyl propanolamine (PPP), a similar drug, increases blood pressure causing confusion, stroke, hallucinations and psychotic behaviour.

- *Special clothing and body wraps:* These help 'weight loss in specific spots' of the body so as to reduce body size. The small weight loss that occurs is the result of temporary water loss due to application of heat and vibrations.

- *Surgery:* Surgical techniques such as jaw wiring, liposuction and intestinal bypass are used for severely obese persons and may result in side effects.

Obesity management: Strategies for success

- Do not set very high goals. Target a reasonable weight loss of ½ - 1 kg per week.
- Adapt family meals to specific needs by adjusting method of preparation and reducing addition of fats.
- Avoid binges. If you overeat due to social pressures, adjust other meals of the day or of the next day.
- While eating outside home, select simply prepared items rather than combination dishes. Avoid fried foods, select fruits as desserts rather than halwas, ice-creams, puddings, etc.
- Spread food throughout the day to meet energy needs.
- Follow a gradual approach to exercise to get the most benefits.
- Exercise regularly at a comfortable pace.
- Select varied exercises that you enjoy and those that fit your personality and your work schedule.
- Encourage your family and friends to support you and join you in your activity. It is best to inculcate healthy habits in your children when they are young.
- Challenge yourself. Set short-term and long-term goals and celebrate every success.
- Do not be discouraged by plateaus. They often occur after some weight loss. Get started again by increasing your exercise.

Weight Management: Underweight

When you eat more calories than you need to perform your day's activities, your body stores the extra calories and you gain weight. But the problem of underweight is not as simple. Most often, underweight is due to an accompanying disorder. The underlying cause of underweight must be dealt with as a first priority. A wasting disease or malabsorption disorder requires treatment. Activity should be modified and psychological counselling should be started if necessary. Nutritional support and dietary changes are effective along with or after the treatment of the underlying disorder, or when the cause of underweight is merely inadequate food intake.

Dietary management

The objectives of dietary modification are:
- To restore body weight to normal.
- To rebuild body tissues and nutrient stores.
- To maintain desirable body weight and a good nutritional status.

Energy: A nutritious high energy diet providing calories over and above the body's requirement will result in weight gain. An increase of about 500 -1000 Cal per day can result in a weight gain of approximately ½ - 1 kg per week. In case of associated fever or gastrointestinal disorders, higher level of calorie intake may be required.

Protein: Liberal intake of high quality protein will help in building up of muscle tissues. A daily protein intake of 1.25-2 g/kg body weight will be required. For example, if your body weight is 60 kg, you should require 75-120 g protein. Easily digestible proteins of high quality such as milk, eggs and a combination of cereals and pulses should be included in the diet of the underweight person.

Carbohydrates: A high carbohydrate intake is necessary to meet the high energy needs. The bulk of the diet, however, should not be increased as it cuts down food intake. Fibre intake should be just enough for regular bowel movement.

Fats: Fats are energy dense and help to reduce bulk but they should only be used in amounts that can be tolerated. Emulsified fats like butter, cream etc. are better tolerated.

Minerals and vitamins: These must be provided in sufficient amounts. Supplements could be necessary in case of associated nutritional deficiencies.

Diet and feeding pattern: The amount of food intake cannot be substantially increased suddenly. The amount of food at each meal and the frequency of meals should be increased gradually. Calorie density of the foods can be increased without increasing bulk by use of sugar, jam, butter, cream, oil, nuts, etc. To increase the protein content of the diet, milk powder, cheese, cottage cheese (paneer), protein concentrates, etc. can be added to liquid milk and other beverages and soups. Favourite foods and snacks given intermittently can stimulate interest in eating.

Counting Calories

A successful weight loss programme depends on maintaining a negative energy balance over a period of time. Only a sound weight loss programme comprising of diet modification (calorie restriction), increase in activity level and behaviour modification can result in permanent weight loss. Similarly, underweight people need to maintain a positive energy balance over a period of time to gain any substantial amount of weight.

Since weight management depends, to a large extent on the number of calories that you consume and the number of calories that you burn, any person interested in managing his/her weight must be able to count his calories, both intake and expenditure.

This chapter has been divided into three sections. The first and second sections provide nutritive value (energy, protein, fat, carbohydrate and fibre) of common ingredients (raw foods) and recipes. The third section gives the energy expenditure in common exercises and sports. These sections will serve as a useful guide for counting your calories – intake and expenditure.

Nutritive value of common ingredients

The following table gives the nutritive value of common ingredients. The nutrients included are: Energy (Cal), Protein (g), Fat (g), Carbohydrate (g) and Crude Fibre (g). All values are given for 100 g of edible portion of foodstuff. The ingredients are divided into food groups: Cereals, Grains and Products, Pulses and Legumes, Leafy and other Vegetables, Roots and Tubers, Nuts and Oilseeds, Fruits, Fishes and other Sea foods, Meat and Poultry, Milk and Milk Products, Fats and Edible Oils, Sugars, Condiments and Spices and Miscellaneous Foodstuffs. Absence of data for any nutrient in the tables indicates the non-availability of authentic figures and not the total absence of the nutrient in the foodstuff.

Nutritive value of common ingredients
(All the values are per 100 g of edible portion)

Foodstuff	Energy (Cal)	Protein (g)	Fat (g)	Carbohydrate (g)	Fibre (g)
Cereals Grains and Products					
Bajra	361	11.6	5.0	67.5	1.2
Barley	336	11.5	1.3	69.6	3.9
Jowar	349	10.4	1.9	72.6	1.6
Maize, dry	342	11.1	3.6	66.2	2.7
Rice, parboiled, milled	346	6.4	0.4	79.0	0.2
Rice, raw, milled	345	6.8	0.5	78.2	0.2
Rice, flakes	346	6.6	1.2	77.3	0.7
Rice, puffed	325	7.5	0.1	73.6	0.3
Wheat, flour (whole)	341	12.1	1.7	69.4	1.9
Wheat, flour (refined)	348	11.0	0.9	73.9	0.3
Wheat, semolina	348	10.4	0.8	74.8	0.2
Wheat, vermicelli	352	8.7	0.4	78.3	0.2
Wheat, bread (brown)	244	8.8	1.4	49.0	1.2
Wheat, bread (white)	245	7.8	0.7	51.9	0.2

Foodstuff	Energy (Cal)	Protein (g)	Fat (g)	Carbohydrate (g)	Fibre (g)
Pulses and Legumes					
Bengal gram, whole	360	17.1	5.3	60.9	3.9
Bengal gram, dal	372	20.8	5.6	59.8	1.2
Bengal gram, roasted	369	22.5	5.2	58.1	1.0
Black gram, dal	347	24.0	1.4	59.6	0.9
Cow pea	323	24.1	1.0	54.5	3.8
Green gram, whole	334	24.0	1.3	56.7	4.1
Green gram, dal	348	24.8	1.2	59.9	0.8
Lentil	343	25.1	0.7	59.0	0.7
Peas, green	093	7.2	0.1	15.9	4.0
Peas, dry	315	19.7	1.1	56.5	4.5
Rajmah	346	22.9	1.3	60.6	4.8
Red gram, dal	335	22.3	1.7	57.6	1.5
Soyabean	432	43.2	19.5	20.9	3.7
Leafy Vegetables					
Amaranth	45	4.0	0.5	6.1	1.0
Bathua leaves	30	3.7	0.4	2.9	0.8
Cabbage	27	1.8	0.1	4.6	1.0
Coriander leaves	44	3.3	0.6	6.3	1.2
Fenugreek leaves	49	4.4	0.9	6.0	1.1
Lettuce	21	2.1	0.3	2.5	0.5

Foodstuff	Energy (Cal)	Protein (g)	Fat (g)	Carbohydrate (g)	Fibre (g)
Mint	48	4.8	0.6	5.8	2.0
Mustard leaves	34	4.0	0.6	3.2	0.8
Radish leaves	28	3.8	0.4	2.4	1.0
Spinach	26	2.0	0.7	2.9	0.6
Roots and Tubers					
Beetroot	43	1.7	0.1	8.8	0.9
Carrot	48	0.9	0.2	10.6	1.2
Colocasia	97	3.0	0.1	21.1	1.0
Onion	59	1.8	0.1	12.6	0.6
Potato	97	1.6	0.1	22.6	0.4
Radish, white	17	0.7	0.1	3.4	0.8
Sweet potato	120	1.2	0.3	28.2	0.8
Turnip	29	0.5	0.2	6.2	0.9
Yam	111	1.4	0.1	26.0	1.0
Other Vegetables					
Ash gourd	10	0.4	0.1	1.9	0.8
Bitter gourd	25	1.6	0.2	4.2	0.8
Bottle gourd	12	0.2	0.1	2.5	0.6
Brinjal	24	1.4	0.3	4.0	1.3
Cauliflower	30	2.6	0.4	4.0	1.2
Cucumber	13	0.4	0.1	2.5	0.4

Foodstuff	Energy (Cal)	Protein (g)	Fat (g)	Carbohydrate (g)	Fibre (g)
Drumstick	26	2.5	0.1	3.7	4.8
French beans	26	1.7	0.1	4.5	1.8
Ghosala	18	1.2	0.2	2.9	2.0
Giant chillies (capsicum)	24	1.3	0.3	4.3	1.0
Jack, tender	51	2.6	0.3	9.4	2.8
Karonda, fresh	42	1.1	2.9	2.9	1.5
Lady's finger	35	1.9	0.2	6.4	1.2
Lotus stem, dry	234	4.1	1.3	51.4	25.0
Plantain, green	64	1.4	0.2	14.0	0.7
Pumpkin fruit	25	1.9	0.1	4.6	0.7
Ridge gourd	17	0.5	0.1	3.4	0.5
Water chestnut, fresh	115	4.7	0.3	23.3	0.6
Nuts and Oilseeds					
Almond	655	20.8	58.9	10.5	1.7
Cashew nut	596	21.2	46.9	22.3	1.3
Chilgoza	615	13.9	49.3	29.0	1.0
Coconut, dry	662	6.8	62.3	18.4	6.6
Coconut, fresh	444	4.5	41.6	13.0	3.6
Gingelly seeds	563	18.3	43.3	25.0	2.9

Foodstuff	Energy (Cal)	Protein (g)	Fat (g)	Carbohydrate (g)	Fibre (g)
Groundnut	567	25.3	40.1	26.1	3.1
Groundnut, roasted	570	26.2	39.8	26.7	3.1
Pistachio nut	626	19.8	53.5	16.2	2.1
Walnut	687	15.6	64.5	11.0	2.6
Water melon seeds	628	34.1	52.6	4.5	0.8
Fruits					
Amla	58	0.5	0.1	13.7	3.4
Apple	59	0.2	0.5	13.4	1.0
Apricot, fresh	53	1.0	0.3	11.6	1.1
Banana, ripe	116	1.2	0.3	27.2	0.4
Cherries, red	64	1.1	0.5	13.8	0.4
Dates, fresh	144	1.2	0.4	33.8	3.7
Grapes, pale green variety	71	0.5	0.3	16.5	2.9
Guava	51	0.9	0.3	11.2	5.2
Jackfruit	88	1.9	0.1	19.8	1.1
Lemon	57	1.0	0.9	11.1	1.7
Litchi	61	1.1	0.2	13.6	0.5
Lime, sweet malta	36	0.7	0.2	7.8	0.6
Lime, sweet mausambi	43	0.8	0.3	9.3	0.5
Loquat	43	0.6	0.3	9.6	0.8
Mango, ripe	74	0.6	0.4	16.9	0.7

Foodstuff	Energy (Cal)	Protein (g)	Fat (g)	Carbohydrate (g)	Fibre (g)
Melon, musk	17	0.3	0.2	3.5	0.4
Melon, water	16	0.2	0.2	3.3	0.2
Orange	48	0.7	0.3	10.9	0.3
Orange juice	9	0.2	0.1	1.9	-
Papaya, ripe	32	0.6	0.1	7.2	0.8
Peaches	50	1.2	0.3	10.5	1.2
Pears	52	0.6	0.2	11.9	1.0
Phalsa	72	1.3	0.9	14.7	1.2
Pineapple	46	0.4	0.1	10.8	0.5
Plum	52	0.7	0.5	11.1	0.4
Pomegranate	65	1.6	0.1	14.5	5.1
Raisins	308	1.8	0.3	74.6	1.1
Raspberry	56	1.0	0.6	11.7	1.0
Sapota	98	0.7	1.1	21.4	2.6
Tomato, ripe	20	0.9	0.2	3.6	0.8
Fish and Other Sea Foods					
Pomfrets, white	87	17.0	1.3	1.8	-
Rohu	97	16.6	1.4	4.4	-
Sardine	101	21.0	1.9	-	-
Singhala	167	20.9	3.1	13.9	-

Foodstuff	Energy (Cal)	Protein (g)	Fat (g)	Carbohydrate (g)	Fibre (g)
Meat and Poultry					
Egg, hen	173	13.3	13.3	–	–
Fowl	109	25.9	0.6	–	–
Goat meat (lean)	118	21.4	3.6	–	–
Liver, sheep	150	19.3	7.5	1.3	–
Mutton, muscle	194	18.5	13.3	–	–
Pork, muscle	114	18.7	4.4	–	–
Milk and Milk Products					
Milk, buffalo's	117	4.3	6.5	5.0	–
Milk, cow's	67	3.2	4.1	4.4	–
Milk, human	65	1.1	3.4	7.4	–
Curd (cow's milk)	60	3.1	4.0	3.0	–
Butter milk	15	0.8	1.1	0.5	–
Skimmed milk, liquid	29	2.5	0.1	4.6	–
Channa, cow's milk	265	18.3	20.8	1.2	–
Channa, buffalo's milk	292	13.4	23.0	7.9	–
Cheese	348	24.1	25.1	6.3	–
Khoya (whole buffalo's milk)	421	14.6	31.2	20.5	–
Khoya (whole cow's milk)	413	20.0	25.9	24.9	–

Foodstuff	Energy (Cal)	Protein (g)	Fat (g)	Carbohydrate (g)	Fibre (g)
Fats and Edible Oils					
Butter	729	–	81.0	–	–
Ghee (cow)	900	–	100	–	–
Hydrogenated oil (fortified)	900	–	100	–	–
Cooking oil	900	–	100	–	–
Sugars					
Sugarcane	398	0.1	0.0	99.4	–
Honey	319	0.3	0.0	79.5	–
Jaggery (cane)	383	0.4	0.1	95.0	–
Sago	351	0.2	0.2	87.1	–
Miscellaneous					
Biscuits, salted	534	6.6	32.4	54.6	–
Biscuits, sweet	450	6.4	15.2	71.9	–
Coconut water	24	1.4	0.1	4.4	–
Makhana	347	9.7	0.1	76.9	–
Papad	288	18.8	0.3	52.4	–
Poppy seeds	408	21.7	19.3	36.8	8.0
Sugarcane juice	39	0.1	0.2	9.1	–
Yeast, dried	344	35.7	1.8	46.3	–

Source: Nutritive Value of Indian Foods, National Institute of Nutrition (NIN), 1996 (Reprint).

Nutritive value of common recipes

Since what you consume are recipes, it is important to know the nutritive value of recipes. The following table gives nutritive values of commonly consumed recipes. The nutrients included are: Energy (Cal), Protein (g), Fat (g), Carbohydrate (g) and Crude Fibre (g). All values are per serving of the recipe. The recipes are divided into the following groups: Beverages, Breakfast Cereals, Eggs, Soups and Sauces, Cereals, Pulses, Meats, Vegetables and Paneer, Salads, Raitas, Desserts, Snacks, Sandwiches, Cakes, Biscuits and Pastries.

Nutritive value of common recipes
(All the values are per serving of the recipe)

Recipe	Size of serving	Energy (Cal)	Protein (g)	Fat (g)	Carbohydrate (g)	Fibre (g)
Beverages						
Tea	1 cup	37	0.6	1.0	5.7	0
Hot coffee	1 cup	118	1.6	8.1	9.7	0
Cold Coffee (with cream)	1 glass	179	3.9	17	27.7	0
Banana Milk Shake	1 glass	227	6.2	7.5	33.8	0.8
Mango Milk Shake	1 glass	236	6.2	7.7	35.6	0.8
Orange Milk Shake	1 glass	216	6.3	7.7	31.0	0
Flavoured Milk Shake	1 glass	180	5.8	7.4	22.9	0
Squash Fruit Punch	1 glass	436	0.2	0.1	110	0
Lemonade	1 glass	107	0.3	0.3	25.7	0.5
Egg Nog	1 glass	228	9.4	11	22.9	0
Jal Jeera	1 glass	37	0.3	0.03	8.8	0.1
Iced Tea	1 glass	137	0.3	0.3	33.2	0.5
Mintade	1 glass	137	0.3	0.3	33.2	0.5
Canjee	1 glass	12	0.2	0.1	2.7	0.4
Lassi (salted)	1 glass	60	3.1	4.0	3	0

Recipe	Size of serving	Energy (Cal)	Protein (g)	Fat (g)	Carbohydrate (g)	Fibre (g)
Breakfast Cereals						
Cracked Wheat Porridge	1 bowl	290	10.0	10.4	39.7	2.5
Cornflakes with Milk	1 bowl	287	9.9	10.8	38.7	1.2
Semolina Upma	1 bowl	147	2.3	7.7	17.1	0.9
Poha	1 bowl	150	2.8	7.3	20.2	1.5
Moongdal Stuffed Cheela	1 bowl	366	15.3	10.9	51.8	6.9
Eggs						
Boiled Egg	1 egg	88	6.7	6.7	0	0
Poached Egg	1 egg	161	6.7	14.8	0	0
Scrambled Egg	1 egg	178	7.3	15.8	0.8	0
French Omelette	1 egg	161	6.7	14.8	0	0
Cheese and Mushroom Omelette	1 egg	295	12.9	27.1	3	0
Soups and Sauces						
Minestrone Soup	1 bowl	89	1.4	5.2	9.4	1.2
Chicken Sweet Corn Soup	1 bowl	327	25.5	13.5	24.6	6.0
Tomato Soup	1 bowl	82	2.1	4.5	8.3	2.3
Green Pea Soup	1 bowl	185	9.0	6.4	23.1	2.2
Spinach Soup	1 bowl	162	3.9	8.9	16.2	5.9
Mixed Vegetable Soup	1 bowl	146	3.3	9.2	12.5	1.4
Cheese Soup	1 bowl	78	0.5	6.5	4.4	0.6

Recipe	Size of serving	Energy (Cal)	Protein (g)	Fat (g)	Carbohydrate (g)	Fibre (g)
Mulligatawny Soup	1 bowl	164	6.1	4.4	24.9	2.6
Cream of Tomato Soup	1 bowl	246	5.4	16.6	18.5	2.3
Cream of Carrot Soup	1 bowl	252	4.6	16.2	21.5	2.0
Cream of Spinach Soup	1 bowl	310	8.5	23.2	16.0	5.1
Cream of Pea Soup	1 bowl	343	12.4	18.2	32.2	2.6
Cream of Mixed Vegetable Soup	1 bowl	263	7.5	13.4	28.0	3.2
Cream of Mushroom Soup	1 bowl	310	6.6	22.4	19.9	0.7
Hot and Sour Soup	1 bowl	183	11.2	9.3	13.2	1.6
Cereals						
Chapattis	3-4	273	9.7	1.4	55.5	5.6
Plain Paranthas	3 medium	363	9.7	11.4	55.5	5.6
Potato Stuffed Parantha	3 medium	631	11.2	31.5	75.8	7.9
Cauliflower Parantha	3 medium	577	12.0	31.7	60.9	7.1
Radish Parantha	3 medium	573	10.8	31.5	61.8	8.2
Dal Parantha	3 medium	664	16.2	33.1	75.6	9.0
Paneer Parantha	3 medium	712	20.9	43.9	58.5	5.9
Methi Parantha	3 medium	651	14.2	32.4	75.8	8.1
Poories (10g oil)	3 medium	375	9.2	12.1	57.4	4.0
Pea Kachories (5g oil)	2	214	6.9	7.4	30.2	1.8
Khasta Kachori (11g oil)	2	441	11.4	18.9	56.3	3.2

Recipe	Size of serving	Energy (Cal)	Protein (g)	Fat (g)	Carbohydrate (g)	Fibre (g)
Nan	1	199	6.7	2.1	38.5	1.5
Bhatura	2-3	176	5.6	3.8	29.9	1.2
Pizza	1	349	18.9	18.9	32.9	2.3
Pancakes	3	228	6.3	12.2	23.4	0.8
Boiled Rice	1 full plate	277	6.0	0.8	61.4	3.6
Mixed Vegetable Pulao	1 full plate	523	17.6	9.0	92.9	7.2
Pea Pulao	1 full plate	510	12.1	9.1	94.8	8.1
Chana Dal and Vegetable Pulao	1 full plate	529	15.1	10.1	94.3	8.5
Paneer Pulao	1 full plate	520	13.3	20.4	70.9	4.3
Chicken Pulao	1 full plate	667	27.9	30.5	68.7	4.3
Mexican Rice	1 full plate	562	22.5	21.8	68.9	5.6
Idli	3-4	156	6.7	0.5	31.5	2.5
Plain Dosa	2	261	7.1	4.6	47.8	3.2
Masala Dosa	1	208	3.0	4.2	39.5	4.5
Mixed Vegetable Dosa	1	183	4.8	4.4	31.2	4.2
Uttapam	2	316	7.8	8.7	51.6	3.9
Beans and Macaroni	1 plate	335	12.1	16.8	38.0	3.7
Macaroni Cheese Pie	1 small casserole dish	392	12.8	17.6	48.8	2.9

Recipe	Size of serving	Energy (Cal)	Protein (g)	Fat (g)	Carbohydrate (g)	Fibre (g)
Meat and Macaroni Casserole	1 small casserole dish	667	27.9	27.4	77.0	6.1
Chicken Chowmein	1 shallow dish	547	31.4	24.2	49.6	3.9
Dal Moong (basic recipe)	1 curry bowl	104	7.3	0.4	17.9	2.6
Chana Dal with Vadi	1 curry bowl	118	1.7	19.1	3.4	27.0
Moong Dal with Vadi (moong dal-8g) (2g-oil)	1 curry bowl	150	9.3	2.5	22.7	3.3
Sambar	1 curry bowl	119	5.6	2.5	18.4	3.2
Green Gram Whole (basic recipe)	1 bowl	100	7.2	0.4	17.0	1.2
Urad Sabut Special	1 bowl	373	9.2	26.8	23.8	2.9
Dry Khatta Chana	1 bowl	232	5.9	11.7	25.6	4.8
Rajmah Curry	1 bowl	268	10.5	11.0	31.8	3.7
Lobia Curry	1 bowl	259	10.9	10.9	29.3	2.8
Besan Gatte Curry	1 bowl	496	21.3	30.6	34.0	5.5
Besan Kadhi with Pakories	1 bowl	228	9.9	10.2	24.1	3.7
Meats						
Keema Matar	1 serving	411	26.9	23.7	22.6	2.8
Mutton do Piaza	1 serving	457	27.0	28.2	24.8	3.2

Recipe	Size of serving	Energy (Cal)	Protein (g)	Fat (g)	Carbohydrate (g)	Fibre (g)
Mutton Korma	1 serving	435	24.0	34.7	7.7	0.8
Palak Meat	1 serving	375	19.1	28.4	10.6	5.2
Shahi Keema Kofta Curry	1 serving	508	23.8	41.3	10.2	1.5
Boti Kebab	1 serving	361	23.6	27.8	5.0	0.5
Mutton Seekh Kebab	1 serving	197	18.6	13.4	0.6	0
Shammi Kebab	1 serving	435	25.0	25.8	25.8	3.6
Nargisi Kofta Curry	1 serving	551	28.3	41.4	16.0	2.5
Tandoori Chicken	1 serving	283	25.8	18.8	0.6	0
Butter Chicken	1 serving	843	35.0	68.0	20.0	3.0
Chilli Chicken	1 serving	472	27.3	35.5	8.8	1.9
Chicken Sweet and Sour	1 serving	430	27.0	33.3	10.0	1.9
Chicken Korma	1 serving	500	28.1	36.4	13.2	2.1
Bengal Fish Curry	1 serving	296	18.4	17.5	16.3	1.6
Tandoori Fish	1 serving	174	25.7	6.8	2.4	0
Tali Machchi	1 serving	378	26.7	19.1	24.8	2.9
Prawn Curry	1 serving	342	30.1	19.9	10.5	2.7
Fish Soufflé	1 serving	403	29.1	23.5	18.6	0.4
Vegetables and Paneer						
Pea Potato Curry	1 bowl	266	8.9	10.3	34.6	4.1
Pea Paneer Curry	1 bowl	349	17.3	20.8	23.6	2.8
Potato Curry	1 bowl	222	2.5	10.2	29.9	3.6

Recipe	Size of serving	Energy (Cal)	Protein (g)	Fat (g)	Carbohydrate (g)	Fibre (g)
Egg Curry	1 bowl	313	15.5	17.6	23.3	2.8
Dahi Aloo	1 bowl	260	4.2	12.2	33.4	3.9
Ghia Kofta Curry	(3-4koftas)	272	3.6	20.9	17.5	2.9
Kela Kofta Curry	(3-4koftas)	273	3.3	15.5	30.1	3.1
Potato Kofta Curry	(3-4koftas)	290	2.9	15.3	35.1	4.1
Paneer Kofta Curry	1 bowl	382	11.2	30.7	15.5	1.5
Aloo Methi	1 bowl	222	5.8	11	24.7	4.1
Sarson ka Saag	1 bowl	156	8.5	6.7	15.7	3.2
Palak Paneer	1 bowl	239	11.2	17.5	9.4	7.7
Dry Arbi (fried)	1 bowl	253	3.6	15.2	25.6	1.6
Masala Arbi	1 bowl	187	3.0	10.1	21.1	1.0
Baingan Bharta	1 small bowl	192	2.8	15.5	10.4	4.5
Bhindi cooked	1 bowl	192	2.6	15	11	6.3
Stuffed Karela (dry)	3 pieces	155	1.3	15.2	3.4	1.8
Kathal (dry)	1 bowl	299	2.2	20.3	27.0	7.1
Mixed Vegetables (Cauliflower, Peas and Potato)	1 bowl	196	5.1	10.3	20.7	2.9
Vegetable Jalfrezi	1 bowl	77	1.1	5.1	6.7	1.4
Cauliflower Mussalam	1 portion	130	5.2	5.8	14.3	3.8
Roasted Potatoes	1-2 potatoes	191	2.4	5.0	34.0	3.8

Recipe	Size of serving	Energy (Cal)	Protein (g)	Fat (g)	Carbohydrate (g)	Fibre (g)
Salads						
Russian Salad	1 small bowl	958	19.7	85.6	27.5	3.3
Tossed Green Salad	1 small bowl	152	1.5	12.2	9.2	2.0
Cucumber and Yogurt Salad	1 small plate	28	1.3	1.3	2.9	1.0
Coleslaw	1 small bowl	468	3.7	44.8	12.0	1.8
Frozen Frosty Fruity Salad	1 slice	252	1.1	16.0	30.2	0.6
French Dressing	3/4th cup	722	0.0	80.0	0.4	0.0
Mayonnaise	1 cup	1226	7.1	132	1.3	0.0
Mayonnaise without Egg	1 cup	883	7.7	90.1	11.0	0.0
Raitas						
Tomato Onion Raita	1 bowl	78	3.7	4.1	6.7	0.6
Cucumber Raita	1 bowl	68	3.3	4.1	4.5	0.8
Ghia Raita	1 bowl	66	3.2	4.1	4.3	0.3
Potato Raita	1 bowl	109	3.9	4.1	14.3	1.3
Mint and Peanut Raita	1 bowl	126	6.6	8.2	6.8	0.9
Spinach Raita	1 bowl	143	7.7	8.7	8.5	4.9
Bathua Raita	1 bowl	147	9.3	8.4	8.5	0.4
Sprouted Green Gram Raita	1 bowl	105	5.8	4.1	11.2	1.2
Boondi Raita	1 bowl	225	7.3	15.0	15.0	2.1
Pineapple Raita	1 bowl	66	3.3	4.1	8.4	0.0
Banana Raita	1 bowl	118	3.7	4.1	16.6	0.4
Mango Raita	1 bowl	97	3.4	4.2	11.5	0.5

Recipe	Size of serving	Energy (Cal)	Protein (g)	Fat (g)	Carbohydrate (g)	Fibre (g)
Desserts						
Rice Kheer	1 bowl	256	7.2	8.3	38.3	0.4
Sevian Kheer	1 bowl	274	7.9	9.2	39.2	1.2
Makhana Kheer	1 bowl	266	6.9	11.2	36.0	0.0
Apple Kheer	1 bowl	243	6.5	8.5	35.4	0.6
Phirni	1 dish	256	7.1	8.3	38.8	0.4
Kulfi	1 mould	314	11.2	14.4	35.3	0.0
Carrot Halwa	1 small bowl	471	8.3	24.5	54.5	2.7
Suji Halwa	1 small bowl	379	3.6	23.2	39.1	0.8
Moong Dal Halwa	1 small bowl	545	13.8	28.2	59	2.7
Soft Stirred Custard	1 bowl	264	12.2	14.0	22.7	0.0
Vanilla Ice Cream	1 Ice Cream cup	289	2.3	22.9	18.2	0
Strawberry Ice Cream	1 Ice Cream cup	289	2.3	22.9	18.2	0.0
Chocolate Ice Cream	1 Ice Cream cup	289	2.3	22.9	18.2	0.0
Chocochip Ice Cream	1 Ice Cream cup	289	2.3	22.9	18.2	0.0
Coffee Ice Cream	1 Ice Cream cup	289	2.3	22.9	18.2	0.0

Recipe	Size of serving	Energy (Cal)	Protein (g)	Fat (g)	Carbohydrate (g)	Fibre (g)
Crunchy Butter Scotch	1 cup	431	3.5	33.0	29.5	0.2
Fruit Ice Cream	1 cup	324	2.6	23.0	26.5	0.3
Fruit Delight	½ small mould	200	3.0	11.0	23.5	0.4
Creamy Chocolate Mousse	1 dish	374	6.8	31.7	15.2	0.1
Cold Lemon Soufflé	1 Soufflé dish	535	6.9	41.9	32.3	0.4
Cold Orange Soufflé	1 Soufflé dish	594	7.8	42.0	46.2	1.5
Cold Pineapple Soufflé	1 Soufflé dish	522	6.7	42	30.0	0.0
Cold Vanilla Soufflé	1 Soufflé dish	539	7.3	42.7	30.6	0.0
Cold Chocolate Soufflé	1 Soufflé dish	539	7.3	42.7	30.6	0.0
Trifle Pudding	1 plate	276	7.4	8.9	41.6	0.8
Date and Nut Pie	1 small plate	256	2.5	8.5	43.0	1.8
Hot Orange Soufflé	1 bowl	237	7.1	11.8	24.8	0.1
Hot Lemon Soufflé	1 bowl	221	6.8	11.8	20.8	0.2
Hot Chocolate Soufflé	1 bowl	248	7.3	12.3	26.7	0.2
Hot Vanilla Soufflé	1 bowl	228	7.3	12.3	21.7	0.2
Snacks						
Gulab Jamun	2	330	6.7	12.9	46.6	0.2
Chenna Murki	10 pieces	275	9.3	10.6	35.6	0.0
Rasgullas	2	230	4.3	5.7	40.4	0.0
Rasmalai	1	180	4.0	5.3	29.5	0.0
Plain Burfi	2	276	10.0	13.0	29.8	0.0

Recipe	Size of serving	Energy (Cal)	Protein (g)	Fat (g)	Carbohydrate (g)	Fibre (g)
Chocolate Burfi	2	276	10.0	13.0	29.8	0.0
Cashewnut Burfi	2	166	3.5	7.8	20.3	0.0
Besan Burfi	2	266	5.3	13.9	30.0	2.7
Khoya Laddoo	2	375	10.7	22.2	33.0	1.8
Besan Laddoo	2	286	5.8	16.4	28.7	2.8
Til Laddoo	2	158	3.2	7.2	20.0	0.0
Gujia	2	313	4.8	13.2	43.6	1.3
Peanut Brittle	2	229	5.2	8.1	33.7	0.9
Murmura Chikki	2	140	0.7	0.0	34.0	0.4
Vegetable Pakoras	6	333	7.8	21.9	26.2	5.2
Masala Onion Pakoras	6	343	7.5	21.8	29.1	4.7
Paneer Pakoras	5	425	15.5	32.1	18.6	3.2
Bread Pakoras	5	489	11.8	22.2	60.5	8.6
Egg Pakoras	5	380	13.0	28.4	18.0	3.2
Chicken Pakoras	5	456	22.6	31.8	18.7	3.2
Fish Pakoras	5	373	19.7	22.8	22.2	3.2
Bondas	5	457	10.7	25.8	45.5	6.4
Vegetable Cutlets	2	216	4.6	10.3	26.2	3.0
Sago Cutlets	2	293	1.7	10.2	48.7	2.5
Chirwa Cutlets	2	325	6.8	10.7	50.4	4.0
Egg Cutlets	2	281	9.2	16.9	22.8	2.5

67

Recipe	Size of serving	Energy (Cal)	Protein (g)	Fat (g)	Carbohydrate (g)	Fibre (g)
Fish Cutlets	2	470	19.1	31.6	27.2	2.5
Minced Meat Cutlets	2	387	21.8	23.6	21.9	2.6
Vegetable Samosas	2	246	4.4	12.0	30.2	2.3
Paneer Pea Samosas	2	255	6.2	16.5	20.5	1.1
Keema Samosa	2	264	10.0	17.2	17.3	1.0
Mathri	2	223	2.8	15.3	18.5	0.8
Urad Dal Vada	2	172	7.2	7.9	17.8	2.1
Dal Vada	2	232	10.3	11.9	20.8	2.1
Mint & Coriander Chutney	1 tbsp	19	0.6	0.1	3.4	0.3
Tomato Ginger Chutney	2 tbsp	6	0.3	0.1	1.0	0.3
Sonth Chutney	1 tbsp	23	0.0	0.0	5.7	0.4
Coconut Chutney	2 tbsp	74	1.6	5.9	3.5	1.8
Curd Mint Dip	2 tbsp	34	1.8	2.0	0.5	0.1
Mayonnaise Vegetable Dip	2 tbsp	284	1.6	29.7	2.1	0.2
Sandwiches						
Tomato Cheese	2	262	7.2	11.8	33.3	4.6
Tomato Cucumber	2	231	5.2	8.6	33.1	4.9
Tomato Grilled	4	300	9.6	15.0	34.8	5.0
French Toasted	2	437	14.6	27.6	34.0	4.6
Chicken Walnut	2	492	16.2	33.1	31.4	4.2
Pineapple Cheese	2	274	8.0	13.4	34.9	4.2

Recipe	Size of serving	Energy (Cal)	Protein (g)	Fat (g)	Carbohydrate (g)	Fibre (g)
Rainbow	2-3	328	7.7	19.2	31.9	4.3
Ribbon	2-3	311	8.3	17.6	35.4	5.8
Checkerboard	3	389	8.2	26.7	31.3	5.8
Club	½ club	588	13.8	44.6	33.5	5.0
Cheese Open	2	321	11.7	18.6	31.5	7.4
Cakes						
Sponge Cake	1 piece	177	6.2	4.6	27.8	0.5
Chocolate Cake	1 piece	156	5.5	4.5	23.3	0.3
Swiss Roll						
(lemon curd filling)	2 swiss rolls	312	7.9	10.9	45.4	0.6
Chocolate Swiss Roll	2 swiss rolls	306	6.7	17.7	30.0	0.4
Pineapple Pastry	1 Pastry	280	7.1	13.2	32.9	0.6
Chocolate Pastry	1 Pastry	228	5.5	12.5	23.3	0.3
Black Forest Gateau	1 piece	144	3.1	7.4	16.2	0.2
Plain Cream Cake	1 piece	229	3.2	13.2	24.3	0.4
Chocolate Cake	1 piece	223	3.1	13.1	23.2	0.4
Orange Cake	1 piece	231	3.2	13.2	25.0	0.4
Lemon Cake	1 piece	233	3.3	13.2	25	0.6
Marbled Cake	1 piece	238	3.6	13.7	25.0	0.4
Dundee Cake	1 piece	205	3.4	11.2	22.5	0.5

Recipe	Size of serving	Energy (Cal)	Protein (g)	Fat (g)	Carbohydrate (g)	Fibre (g)
Eggless Cake	1 piece	355	7.4	13.9	50.4	0.6
Biscuits						
Almond	2	142	2.0	6.6	18.6	0.5
Chocolate	2	151	2.0	6.6	21.0	0.5
Orange	1 double	204	2.2	6.8	33.4	0.5
Coffee Drops	1 small	163	2.9	8.3	18.7	0.5
Cherries and Walnut	3	212	3.0	10.0	27.3	0.6
Cheese Straws	4	156	4.4	10.5	11.6	0.5
Pastries						
Fruit Flan	½	300	4.8	16.6	32.4	1.5
Orange Cream Flan	¼	309	5.1	14.8	38.9	0.9
Custard Tarts	2	281	6.8	16.4	26.7	0.9
Jam Tarts	2	269	3.3	12.5	36.0	0.9
Lemon Chiffon Pie	¼	378	5.0	24.1	35.2	0.9
Orange Chiffon Pie	¼	386	5.0	24.1	37.1	0.9
Chocolate Éclairs	2	483	5.6	35.7	34.7	0.6
Cheese Balls	6	290	6.9	25.3	10.9	0.4
Minced Meat Patties	1	390	11.0	29.5	19.3	0.9
Paneer Patties	1	294	7.5	20.5	19.9	1.0

Energy expenditure in physical activity and sports
The stresses of modern urban living have made our lifestyles increasingly sedentary. A little extra calories that we may burn through some exercise can work wonders. Walking briskly for just 30 minutes a day, 3-4 times a week is good enough, good for your body weight, good for your heart.

The number of calories that you burn in any physical activity or sports depends upon your body weight and on the intensity of the workout, that is, on how vigorously you perform the exercise. Energy expenditure in various physical activities and sports is listed in the table below. The activities are divided into: Gym Activities, Training and Sport Activities, Outdoor Activities, Home and Daily Life Activities and Occupational Activities. The values are given for body weights ranging from 60 kg to 100 kg. Wherever possible, variation in intensity of activity has been included. All values are given as calories per minute. To find out the number of calories that you burn in your workout, select the activity and read the value across your body weight and multiply by the time in minutes that you spend in the activity.

Energy expenditure in physical activity & sports
(All values are given in calories per minute)

Activity	60 kg	70 kg	80 kg	90 kg	100 kg	110 kg
Gym Activities						
Aerobics: low impact	6	7	8	8	10	11
Aerobics: high impact	7	9	10	11	12	14
Bicycling, Stationary, moderate	7	9	10	11	12	14
Bicycling, Stationary, vigorous	11	13	15	16	18	20
Stepping	6	7	8	9	11	12
Stretching, yoga	4	5	6	6	7	8
Weight lifting	3	4	4	5	5	6

Activity	60 kg	70 kg	80 kg	90 kg	100 kg	110 kg
Training and Sports Activities						
Badminton	5	6	6	7	8	9
Basketball	8	8	11	12	14	15
Billiards	3	3	4	4	4	5
Bicycling: 12-13.9 mph	8	10	11	12	14	15
Bicycling: 14-15.9 mph	11	12	14	15	18	19
Bicycling: 16-19 mph	13	15	17	18	21	23
Bicycling: > 20 mph	17	20	23	25	29	32
Bowling	3	4	4	5	5	6
Boxing	10	11	13	14	16	17
Dancing	6	7	8	8	10	11
Football	8	10	11	12	14	15
Golf	6	7	8	8	10	11
Gymnastics	4	5	6	6	7	8
Hockey	8	10	11	12	14	15
Rope jumping	11	12	14	15	18	19
Running: 5 mph	8	10	11	12	14	15
Running: 6 mph	11	12	14	15	18	19
Running: 7.5 mph	13	15	18	19	22	24
Running: 10 mph	17	20	23	25	29	32
Soccer	7	9	10	11	12	14
Swimming: general	6	7	8	9	11	12
Swimming: backstroke	8	10	11	12	14	15
Swimming: breaststroke	11	12	14	15	18	19
Swimming: butterfly	12	14	15	17	19	21
Tennis	7	9	10	11	12	14
Walk: 3.5 mph	4	5	6	6	7	8
Walk: 4 mph	5	6	6	7	8	9
Walk: 4.5 mph	5	6	7	8	9	10
Wrestling	6	7	8	9	11	12
Outdoor Activities						
Gardening	5	6	6	7	8	9
Mowing lawn	6	6	8	8	10	11
Home & Daily Life Activities						
Child care: bathing, feeding, etc.	4	4	5	5	6	7
Cooking	3	3	4	4	4	5
Food shopping	4	4	5	5	6	7
Moving	4	4	5	5	6	7
Playing with kids	4	5	6	6	7	8
Reading: sitting	1	1	2	2	2	2
Standing in line	1	2	2	2	2	2
Sleeping	1	1	1	1	1	1
Watching TV	1	1	1	1	1	1

Activity	60 kg	70 kg	80 kg	90 kg	100 kg	110 kg
Occupational Activities						
Bartending/Server	3	3	4	4	4	5
Carpentry work	4	4	5	5	6	7
Coaching sports	4	5	6	6	7	8
Coal mining	6	7	8	9	11	12
Computer work	1	2	2	2	2	3
Construction, general	6	7	8	8	10	11
Desk work	2	2	2	3	3	3
Driving	2	2	3	3	4	4
Fire fighting	13	15	17	18	21	23
Heavy tools	8	10	11	12	14	15
Light office work	2	2	2	2	3	3
Police officer	3	3	4	4	4	5
Sitting in class	2	2	2	3	3	3
Sitting in meetings	2	2	2	2	3	3
Welding	3	4	4	5	5	6

Tips for Controlling Calorie Intake

While controlling calorie intake is the most crucial aspect of any weight reduction programme, it does not imply that the person concerned must forego his taste buds. You can limit your calories without compromising on taste. This chapter will provide you tips on controlling calorie intake including low calorie cooking methods and recipes. It will also provide information on low calorie alternatives to high calorie foods, role of fibre and some high fibre recipes, artificial sweeteners and fat replacers.

Low calorie cooking methods

Steaming: Steaming is cooking food by surrounding it with steam produced by boiling water. Food can be cooked by *direct steaming* in which the food is placed in a perforated basket and kept covered over boiling water. In *indirect steaming,* food is placed in a covered dish which is put in steam or over boiling water. *Pressure cooking* is a form of steaming in which water is boiled under high pressure. Steaming is an excellent no-fat method of cooking. The water can be scented with herbs or spices to impart flavour. Steaming is commonly used for cooking fish, idli, dhokla, puddings and custards and vegetables like cabbage, peas, beans and carrots.

Boiling: Boiling is cooking food in boiling water. Cooking is done in a covered pan of correct size using minimum water to cover the food.

Roasting: Roasting means cooking uncovered in a hot air oven. Roasting intensifies flavour. It is generally used for high quality tender meats, chicken, vegetables, potato, tomato, brinjal, cereals, semolina, broken wheat, vermicelli etc.

Sautéing: Sautéing means frying and tossing food in a small amount of hot fat in a shallow frying pan. Pieces should be of the same size for even cooking. Vegetables like cabbages, beans, carrots, capsicums, bean sprouts, onions, tomatoes, noodles and thin sections of meat are commonly cooked by sautéing. Vegetables can be steamed before sautéing them in a small amount of fat. Less fat is consumed in this cooking process.

Stewing: Stewing is cooking food slowly in a covered pan using a small quantity of liquid which is kept simmering (not boiling). This technique makes the food tender using minimal fat. It is commonly applied to meat, chicken, fruits and vegetables.

Grilling: Grilling is cooking food by direct or radiant heat under a grill, over an open fire or burning coals. This type of cooking imparts a smoky flavour. Grilling is generally used as a final step to brown dishes. Grilling is commonly used for tender meat, steaks, chops, fish, liver, kidney, chicken, vegetables, stuffed tomatoes, capsicum, cauliflower, bottle gourd etc.

Poaching: Poaching means cooking food in a minimum of water that is kept gently simmering (not boiling). Adding spices or herbs to the liquid imparts flavour. Egg and fish are commonly poached.

Braising: Braising is a combined method of roasting and stewing. To braise means to brown meat and vegetables in a minimal amount of fat and subsequently to cover and cook in a small amount of simmering liquid. This technique makes tender sturdy vegetables and tough cuts of meat.

Marinate: To marinate means to soak food (usually meats) in a mixture of vinegar, oil, spices, curd and lime. The meat is usually steeped in the above mixture (called marinade) before it is cooked in order to improve the flavour and make it more tender. Oils can be added if desired. Soya, ginger and garlic can be added to the marinade for an Asian-style dish and tomatoes for an Italian touch.

Low calorie recipes

1. Minestrone soup

Number of serving: 1
Size of serving: 1 bowl

Ingredients

Onion	:	20 g
Garlic	:	½ clove
Carrot	:	20 g
Bay leaf	:	1
Cabbage	:	5 g
Spaghetti	:	5 g
Tomato	:	30 g
Salt	:	½ teaspoon
Stock	:	1 ½ cups
Pepper	:	a dash
Oil	:	5 g

Procedure

1. Chop the onion, shred the cabbage and dice the carrots.
2. Heat oil in a saucepan; add the onion and the carrot and sauté.
3. Add the stock and bring to a boil. Add the macaroni, skinned and chopped tomato and bay leaf.
4. Simmer gently for 20 minutes. Add the cabbage and seasoning.
5. Cook till the vegetables are soft.
6. Serve hot, garnished with grated cheese.

Nutritive value per serving: 89 Cal, 1.4 g protein, 5.2 g fat, 9.4 g carbohydrate, 1.2 g fibre.

2. Carrot Appetizer (Canjee)

Number of serving: 6
Size of serving: 1 glass

Ingredients

Black carrots	: 50 g
Water	: 4 cups
Mustard seeds, coarsely ground	: 10 g
Salt	: ½ teaspoon
Chilli powder (optional)	: ¼ teaspoon

Procedure

1. Wash, scrape and cut the carrots into 8 cm long, thin pieces.
2. Add the carrots and other ingredients to water. Mix well.
3. Store in earthenware pots or glass jar.
4. Put in the sun for 7 days or more to sour.

5. Serve in a medium-size glass over crushed ice.
Nutritive value per serving: 12 Cal, 0.2 g protein, 0.1 g fat, 2.7 g carbohydrate, 0.4 g fibre.

3. Jellied sunshine fruit salad
Number of serving: 1
Size of serving: 1 small mould

Ingredients

Gelatine	:	1 teaspoon
Cold water	:	½ tablespoon
Hot water	:	¼ cup
Pineapple	:	40 g
Lemon juice	:	½ tablespoon
Vinegar	:	¼ tablespoon
Salt	:	1/8 teaspoon
Carrot, grated	:	50 g
Walnut, chopped	:	1
Pineapple syrup	:	2 tablespoons
Lettuce	:	2 leaves

Procedure

1. Soak the gelatine in cold water and heat to dissolve.
2. Drain the pineapple, reserve its syrup. Cut the slices into tiny pieces.
3. Add water to the syrup to make ¼ cup. Add to the gelatine with the lemon juice, vinegar and salt. Chill till partly set.
4. Fold in the pineapple bits, walnuts and carrots.
5. Pour it into a small jelly mould. Chill till firm.
6. Serve chilled unmoulded on greens/lettuce leaves.
Nutritive value per serving: 33 Cal, 0.8 g protein, 0.2 g fat, 10.6 g carbohydrate, 1.1 g fibre.

4. Corn muffins

Number of serving: 1
Size of serving: 1 muffin

Ingredients

Corn meal	:	5 g
Wheat flour	:	8 g
Bengal gram flour	:	5 g
Salt	:	a pinch
Baking powder	:	¼ teaspoon
Baking soda	:	a pinch
Egg white	:	10 g
Curd	:	10 g
Water	:	¾ teaspoon
Carrots	:	5 g

Procedure

1. Sift the corn meal, wheat flour, bengal gram flour, salt, baking powder and soda together.
2. Make a batter with egg, curd and water. Fold in the grated carrots.
3. Pour into a muffin mould and bake at 350°F for 20 minutes.

Nutritive value per serving: 76 Cal, 2.7 g protein, 1.1 g fibre.

5. Grape and orange whip

Number of serving: 2
Size of serving: 1 orange case

Ingredients:

Orange	: 150 g/1 large
Orange flavoured jelly crystals	: 15 g
Water	: 30 ml

Cream, whipped	: 15 g/1 tablespoon
Egg white	: ½
Grapes	: 30 g

Procedure:

1. Halve the orange carefully. Crimp the edges. Squeeze out the juice but keep the orange cases intact.
2. Dissolve the jelly crystals in 2 tablespoon hot water. Let it cool a little, then add orange juice to make 3/8 cup (add water if required).
3. Allow to cool in the fridge (not in the freezer) till it begins to stiffen slightly.
4. Whisk the cream, whisk the egg white stiffly and fold these in the semi-stiffened mixture.
5. Put a layer of deseeded grapes at the bottom of each orange case, reserve some grapes for decoration. Top with jelly mixture and let it set in the fridge (not in freezer).
6. Serve decorated with halved grapes.

Nutritive value per serving: 76 Cal, 1.6 g protein, 2.7 g fat, 11.5 g carbohydrate, 1.3 g fibre.

6. Raspberry sparkle

Number of serving: 1
Size of serving: 1 mould

Ingredients

Orange	: 150 g
Skimmed milk	: 60 ml
Gelatine	: 5 g
Raspberries	: 20 g
Sweetex	: 1 drop

Procedure

1. Boil milk with half the gelatine and add sweetex. Put into a jelly mould and set.
2. Extract juice out of orange. Heat juice with gelatine and cool.
3. When milk is set, pour the juice over it.
4. Put stewed raspberries into the orange juice when it is half set.
5. Set in a refrigerator.
6. Garnish with halved raspberries, after unmoulding.

Nutritive value per serving: 58 Cal, 2 g fat, 4 g carbohydrate.

7. Fruity tarts

Number of serving: 4

Size of serving: 1 tart

Ingredients

Buckwheat flour	:	20 g
Soy flour	:	20 g
Maize flour	:	20 g
Curd	:	40 g
Apple	:	40 g
Papaya	:	40 g
Guava	:	40 g
Egg white	:	60 g
Baking powder	:	1 teaspoon
Lemon juice	:	1 teaspoon
Green gram, sprouted	:	20 g

Procedure

1. Roast soy flour and mix with buckwheat flour and maize flour.
2. Add baking powder and strain juice.
3. Beat egg white to a stiff stage and fold into the flour.

4. Using curd, knead the flour into soft dough.
5. Roll out, cut into round, and line tart moulds.
6. Bake in a moderate oven till done (15-20 minutes).
7. Dice fruits and add lemon juice and spread out.
8. Fill tartlets with fruits and sprout mixture.

Nutritive value per serving: 82 Cal, 5.6 g protein, 1.3 g fat, 10.6 g carbohydrate.

Fibre - The wonder non-nutrient

Dietary fibres are constituents of plants that are resistant to digestion in the human digestive tract. The types of fibre – soluble and insoluble, their functions and sources have been discussed earlier in this book. The table below gives fibre content of common foods.

Total fibre content of common foods
(Values in g/100 g edible portion)

High (> 10)	Medium (1 - 10)	Low (< 1)	Nil
Wheat	Rice	Refined and	Sugar
Jowar	Most vegetables	processed foods	Fats/oils
Bajra	Most fruits		Milk
Ragi	Coconut		All types of meat
Maize	Sesame (til)		
Legumes			
Pulses &			
Legumes			

A fibre rich diet helps in weight management in many ways. Fibre rich foods are generally 'calorie poor'. They also contribute bulk to our diet and hence give a sensation of fullness of stomach, early satiety and very few calories. They also delay gastric emptying and hunger sensation and increase inter-meal hunger interval besides decreasing insulin (appetite-stimulant) levels.

Low calorie alternatives to high calorie foods

High calorie food		Low calorie food	
Food item	Calories	Food item	Calories
Full cream milk	170 Cal/glass	Skimmed milk	10 Cal/200 ml
Aerated drinks	60-80 Cal/200 ml	Fresh lime juice	40 Cal/glass
Lassi (sweet)	250 Cal/glass	Plain buttermilk	40 Cal/glass
Lassi (salty)	180 Cal/glass	Plain buttermilk	40 Cal/glass
Sherbat	80 Cal/glass	Plain buttermilk	40 Cal/bowl
Thick cream soup	200 Cal/bowl	Clear soup	70 Cal
Parantha	200 Cal	Plain chapatti	80 Cal/cup
Pulao/ Fried rice	170 Cal/cup	Boiled rice	80 Cal/cup
Biryani	300 Cal/serving	Boiled rice	70 Cal/cup
Fried vegetables	150 Cal/cup	Steamed vegetables	45-80/serving
Coleslaw salad	175 Cal/serving	Sprouts or vegetable salad	40-50 Cal/serving
Regular pudding or dessert	150 Cal/serving	Fresh fruit with jelly	60 Cal/serving
Fried egg/omelette	120 Cal/serving	Boiled/poached egg	negligible
Oil-based dressing	90 Cal/tablespoon	Lemon dressing	265 Cal/100 g
Malai paneer	620 Cal/100 g	Low fat cottage cheese	29/100 ml
Cream (25 % fat)	225 Cal/100 g	Skimmed milk	
Vegetable sandwich with butter	300 Cal/sandwich	Vegetable sandwich without butter	200 Cal/sandwich
French fries	350 Cal/serving	Boiled/roasted potato	150 Cal/serving
Fried cashew nuts	800 Cal/serving	Roasted grams	370 Cal/100 g
Fried peanuts	750 Cal/serving	Roasted grams	370 Cal/100 g
Roasted cashewnuts	600 Cal/serving	Roasted grams	370 Cal/100 g
Roasted peanuts	570 Cal/serving	Roasted grams	370 Cal/100 g

Hence, a high-fibre, low-fat diet is ideal for sustained weight loss. Along with a regular exercise schedule, a high-fibre, low-fat diet provides the key to weight reduction and positive health. Given below are some high-fibre recipes containing bran.

1. Wheat bran biscuits (sweet)
Number of serving: 8
Size of serving: 3 biscuits

Ingredients

Wheat bran	:	100 g
Wheat flour refined (maida)	:	100 g
Oil/ghee	:	50 g
Jaggery	:	100 g

Procedure
1. Beat fat till creamy.
2. Add flour, wheat bran, crushed caramelised jaggery and make dough. Keep it for 4-5 hours.
3. Roll out and cut into required shapes
4. Bake at 350° F for 25-30 minutes or until done.

Nutritive value per serving: 120 Cal, 4 g fibre.

2. Wheat bran biscuits (salty)
Number of serving: 8
Size of serving: 3 biscuits

Ingredients

Wheat bran	:	100 g
Wheat flour refined (maida)	:	100 g
Oil/ghee	:	50 g
Curd	:	100 g

Thyme and salt to taste

Procedure
1. Beat fat till creamy.
2. Add curd and mix well.
3. Add flour, wheat bran, salt and thyme and knead to make dough. Keep it for 4-5 hours.
4. Roll out and cut into required shapes
5. Bake at 350° F for 25-30 minutes or until done.

Nutritive value per serving: 95 Cal, 4 g fibre.

3. Bran chapatti
Number of serving: 1
Size of serving: 4 chapattis

Ingredients

Wheat flour whole	: 60 g
Wheat bran	: 20 g

Procedure
1. Make dough of wheat flour and bran with water. Leave for about half an hour.
2. Divide the dough into 4 balls and roll out the balls into chapattis.
3. Cook the chapattis.

Nutritive value per serving: 270 Cal.

4. Yogurt and Lentil Patties (Dahi vada)
Number of serving: 6
Size of serving: 2 vadas

Ingredients:

Black gram dal (washed)	:25 g
Curd	:250 g
Wheat bran	:100 g
Salt to taste	

Black pepper to taste
Roasted cumin seeds
(jeera)   :1 tsp
Ginger   :1" piece

Procedure
1. Soak dal overnight.
2. Grind dal, bran and ginger together to thick batter consistency.
3. Make balls and fry them.
4. Beat curd, add roasted jeera powder and salt and pepper to taste.
5. Soak vadas in water, squeeze and soak them in curd.

Nutritive value per serving: 125 Cal.

Artificial sweeteners

A variety of artificial sweeteners have been tested and approved for use. Artificial sweeteners are of two types-nutritive and non-nutritive. Nutritive sweeteners include sorbitol and fructose; these sweeteners provide calories and should be used with discretion.

Non-nutritive sweeteners include aspartame, saccharin, cyclamates, acesulfame K etc. *Aspartame* is a low calorie sweetener, about 200 times sweeter than sugar. It is virtually calorie-free and can be consumed in amounts upto 40 mg per kilogram of body weight. It is considered safe for consumption by all individuals except for persons suffering from phenylketonuria. *Saccharin* is a calorie-free sweetener which is 300-500 times sweeter than sugar. The acceptable daily intake for saccharin is 5.0 mg per kilogram of body weight. *Cyclamate* is also a calorie-free sweetener 30 times sweeter than sugar. It can be consumed in amounts upto 11 mg per kilogram of body weight. *Acesulfame K* is

130-200 times sweeter than sugar and is calorie-free. The acceptable daily intake for acesulfame K has been set at 15 mg per kilogram of body weight.

Fat replacers

Fat replacers are substances that can be used to replace some or all of the fat in food products. They have the potential to help consumers reduce total fat consumption and hence, indirectly reduce total calorie consumption. Because fat replacers can improve both the taste and texture of lower-fat foods, they can help alleviate the sense of deprivation that can impede compliance with a low-fat, low-calorie diet. Fat replacers are of three types:

Carbohydrate based fat replacers: These include cellulose, maltodextrins, gums, starches, fibres, polydextrose, etc. Carbohydrate based fat replacers are much lower in calories than fat. Although they are heat stable for baking, they do not melt and so cannot be used for sautéing or frying.

Protein based fat replacers: These are generally based on egg whites, whey, protein or soya. Their texture, appearance and mouth-feel make them particularly suited for use in dairy products. Although they are suitable for heat applications such as baking, they cannot be used for frying.

Fat based fat replacers: These are based on fat, usually vegetable oils. The fatty acids in the vegetable oils are chemically treated so that they provide few or no calories. Fat based fat replacers have the advantage of heat stability and can be used in frying.

All these fat replacers should be available in India shortly. Fruit and vegetable purees can also be used as fat replacers. Apple sauce, banana puree, puree of others fruits and vegetables can be used for replacing fat in baked goods and sauces. These purees and sauces provide some of the moisture, volume and texture of fats, besides providing varying amounts of fibres, vitamins and minerals.

Nutrition– Myths and Facts

Myth: Starvation and rapid decrease in body weight are good.

Fact: Reduction in body weight should be gradual, starvation is not the solution.

Myth: One meal a day is good for body weight reduction.

Fact: Frequent and small meals are far better and more useful.

Myth: A zero-fat diet is excellent.

Fact: Some amount of fat is necessary.

Myth: Only fat intake needs to be reduced for reducing weight.

Fact: A total change towards a healthy diet and healthy lifestyle is necessary.

Myth: Only vigorous exercises are good.

Fact: Even a long brisk walk will help very much.

Myth: Vegetable oils are fat-free, cholesterol-free.

Fact: Vegetable oils are cholesterol free. All plant products are devoid of cholesterol and so are vegetable oils. However, they are not fat-free and excess consumption of vegetable oils can cause an increase in total fat intake and total calorie intake.

Myth: Vegetable oils can be consumed in any amounts.

Fact: Moderation must be exercised in their use.

Appendix I
Recommended Dietary Allowances for Indians

Group	Particulars	Body wt.	Net energy	Protein	Fat	Calcium	Iron
		kg	Cal/d	g/d	g/d	mg/d	mg/d
Man	Sedentary		2425				
	Moderate	60	2875	60	20	400	28
	Heavy		3800				
Woman	Sedentary		1875				
	Moderate	50	2225	50	20	400	30
	Heavy		2925				
	Pregnant	50	+300	+15	30	1000	38
	Lactation						
	0-6 mths.	50	+550	+25	45	1000	30
	6-12 mths.	50	+400	+18	45	1000	30
Infants	0-6 mths.	5.4	108/kg	2.05/kg	-	500	-
	6-12 mths.	8.6	98/kg	1.65/kg	-	500	-

Vitamin A µg/d		Thiamine	Riboflavin	Niacin	Pyrid	Vit. C oxins	Folic acid	Vit. B-12
Ret.	Car.	mg/d	mg/d	mg/d	mg/d	mg/d	µg/d	µg/d
		1.2	1.4	16				
600	2400	1.4	1.6	18	2.0	40	100	1
		1.6	1.9	21				
		0.9	1.1	12				
600	2400	1.1	1.3	14	2.0	40	100	1
		1.2	1.5	16				
600	2400	+0.2	+0.2	+2	2.5	40	400	1
950	3800	+0.3	+0.3	+4	2.5	80	150	1.5
950	3800	+0.2	+0.2	+3	2.5	80	150	1.5
350	1400	55	65	710	0.1	25	25	0.2
		µg/kg	µg/kg	µg/kg				
		50	60	650				
		µg/kg	µg/kg	µg/kg				
350	1400				0.4	25	25	0.2

Ret. – Retinol
Car. – Carotene

Group	Particulars	Body wt.	Net energy	Protein	Fat	Calcium	Iron
		kg	Cal/d	g/d	g/d	mg/d	mg/d
Children	1-3 years	12.2	1240	22			12
	4-6 years	19.0	1690	30	25	400	18
	7-9 years	26.9	1950	41			26
Boys	10-12 years	35. 4	2190	54	25	600	34
Girls	10-12 years	31.5	1970	57	25	600	19
Boys	13-15 years	47.8	2450	70	25	600	41
Girls	13-15 years	46.7	2060	65	25	600	28
Boys	16-18 years	57.1	2640	78	25	500	50
Girls	16-18 years	49.9	2060	63	25	500	20

Vitamin A μg/d		Thiamine	Riboflavin	Niacin	Pyrid	Vit. C oxins	Folic acid	Vit. B-12
Ret.	Car.	mg/d	mg/d	mg/d	mg/d	mg/d	μg/d	μg/d
400	1600	0.6	0.7	8	0.9		30	
400	1600	0.9	1.0	11	0.9	40	40	0.2-
600	2400	1.0	1.2	13	1.6		60	1.0
600	2400	1.1	1.3	15	1.6	40	70	0.2-
600	2400	1.0	1.2	13	1.6	40	70	1.0
600	2400	1.2	1.5	16	2.0	40	100	0.2-
600	2400	1.0	1.2	14	2.0	40	100	1.0
600	2400	1.3	1.6	17	2.0	40	100	0.2-
600	2400	1.0	1.2	14	2.0	40	100	1.0

Ret. – Retinol
Car. – Carotene

Source: Indian Council of Medical Research, 1996 (Reprint)

Glossary

Amla – Indian gooseberry
Arbi – colocasia
Baingan bharta – mashed brinjals
Bajra – pearl millet
Bathua leaves – Chenopodium album
Besan gatte curry – gram flour gravy
Besan kadhi with pakories – gram flour curry with curd and dumplings.
Bhatura – fermented Indian bread
Bhindi cooked – lady's finger preparation
Bonda – mashed potato dumpling
Boondi – fried gram flour balls
Boti kebab – chicken kebab
Burfi – sweet squares
Canjee – carrot appetizer
Chana – bengal gram
Channa – cottage cheese
Chapatti – flat bread
Chenna murki – cottage cheese sweet balls
Chirwa – rice flakes
Dahi aloo – potato with curd
Dal - pulses
Dhokla – bengal gram flour and semolina steam cakes (low calorie)
Dosa – fried rice and black gram preparation (with or without fillings)
Ghia – ghosala
Gujia – fried puffs with sweet fillings
Gulab jamun – rose sweet
Halwa – sweet Indian dessert

Idli – steamed rice and black gram preparation
Jal jeera – cumin drink
Jalfrezi – minced vegetable
Jowar – great millet
Kachori – refined flour puff with savoury filling
Karela – bitter gourd
Karonda – a pea sized vegetable
Kathal – jackfruit
Keema matar – minced meat with peas
Kela – banana
Khasta kachori – fat-rich white flour puff
Khatta channa – bengal gram whole
Kheer – sweet milk-based dessert
Khoya –a sweet dairy product
Korma – fried dumplings in onion sauce
Kulfi – frozen milk-based dessert
Laddoos – sweet balls
Lassi – buttermilk
Litchi – lychee
Lobia – cow pea
Makhana – cereal based puff
Malai – cream
Mathri – fried refined flour snack
Methi - fenugreek
Moongdal stuffed cheela – green gram pancakes
Murmura chikki – puffed rice wafers
Murrabba – fruit pressure
Mussalam – baked cauliflower
Mutton do piaza – mutton with onions
Nan – fermented Indian bread
Nargisi kofta – mince meat and egg dumplings
Pakora – gram flour dumplings with filling
Palak – spinach
Paneer – cheese
Papad – wafer
Parantha – flat bread with ghee
Phalsa – a small fruit
Phirni – ground rice and milk desert
Poha – rice flakes preparation
Poori – puffy white bread

Pulao – fried rice
Ragi – coarse millet
Raita – curd with spices and vegetables and other additions
Rajma – kidney beans
Rasgulla – sweet balls
Rasmalai – milk syrup with sweet balls
Rohu - a fresh water fish
Sambar – red gram gravy with tamarind
Samosa – small, fried Indian pastry turnover with savoury fillings
Sarson ka saag – mustard leaf
Sevian – vermicelli
Shahi keema kofta curry – mince meat dumplings in gravy
Shammi kebab – mutton kebab
Singhala – a type of fish
Sonth Chutney – ground ginger sauce
Suji – semolina
Tali machchi – fried fish
Tandoori – roasted
Til – sesame
Upma – kind of pudding
Urad sabut – black gram whole
Uttapam – dosa with toppings
Vada/Vadi – black gram balls